MULTISYSTEM DISEASES

Other titles in the *New Clinical Applications* Series:

Dermatology (Series Editor Dr J. L. Verbov)
Dermatological Surgery
Superficial Fungal Infections
Talking Points in Dermatology – I
Treatment in Dermatology
Current Concepts in Contact Dermatitis
Talking Points in Dermatology – II
Tumours, Lymphomas and Selected Paraproteinaemias
Relationships in Dermatology
Talking Points in Dermatology – III
Mycobacterial Skin Diseases

Cardiology (Series Editor Dr D. Longmore)
Cardiology Screening

Rheumatology (Series Editors Dr J. J. Calabro and Dr W. Carson Dick)
Ankylosing Spondylitis
Infections and Arthritis
Osteoporosis

Nephrology (Series Editor Dr G. R. D. Catto)
Continuous Ambulatory Peritoneal Dialysis
Management of Renal Hypertension
Chronic Renal Failure
Calculus Disease
Pregnancy and Renal Disorders
Multisystem Diseases
Glomerulonephritis I
Glomerulonephritis II
Haemodialysis
Urinary Tract Infections

NEW
CLINICAL
APPLICATIONS
NEPHROLOGY

MULTISYSTEM DISEASES

Editor

G. R. D. CATTO

DSc, MD, FRCP, (Lond., Edin. and Glasg.)

Professor in Medicine and Therapeutics
University of Aberdeen
UK

KLUWER ACADEMIC PUBLISHERS
DORDRECHT / BOSTON / LONDON

Distributors

for the United States and Canada: Kluwer Academic Publishers, PO Box 358, Accord Station, Hingham, MA 02018–0358, USA
for all other countries: Kluwer Academic Publishers Group, Distribution Center, PO Box 322, 3300 AH Dordrecht, The Netherlands

British Library Cataloguing in Publication Data

Multisystem diseases
1. Man. Kidneys. Diseases
I. Catto, Graeme R.D. (Graeme Robertson Dawson), *1945–*
II. Series
616.6′1

ISBN-13: 978-94-010-7497-1 e-ISBN-13: 978-94-009-2223-5
DOI: 10.1007/978-94-009-2223-5

Published in the United Kingdom by Kluwer Academic Publishers, PO Box 55, Lancaster, UK.

Kluwer Academic Publishers BV incorporates the publishing programmes of D. Reidel, Martinus Nijhoff, Dr W. Junk and MTP Press.

CONTENTS

LIST OF AUTHORS

F. W. Ballardie
Department of Renal Medicine
University of Manchester
Manchester Royal Infirmary
Oxford Road
Manchester M13 9WL
UK

J. J. Bending
District General Hospital
King's Drive
Eastbourne
East Sussex BN21 2UD
UK

S. M. Crawford
Clinical Oncology Unit
University of Bradford
Bradford
West Yorkshire BD7 1DP
UK

H. Keen
Unit for Metabolic Medicine
United Medical and Dental
Schools
Guy's Hospital
London SE1 9RT
UK

R. S. Trompeter
Department of Paediatrics
Royal Free Hospital
Pond Street
Hampstead
London NW3 2QG
UK

SERIES EDITOR'S FOREWORD

During the last decade facilities for treating patients with end-stage renal failure have expanded in all Westernized countries. Partly as a consequence, interest has been stimulated in many multisystem diseases which may progress to chronic renal failure. Some of these diseases such as diabetes mellitus are common but still have controversial aspects to their investigation and management. Others such as lupus nephritis are relatively rare but respond well to recent advances in therapy.

In addition to diabetes mellitus and lupus nephritis this volume has chapters on multiple myeloma and Henoch–Schönlein purpura. All the chapters have been written by acknowledged experts who have emphasized the practical aspects of patient management. The information contained in this volume should thus prove of interest not only to nephrologists but to all practising clinicians.

ABOUT THE EDITOR

Professor Graeme R. D. Catto is Professor in Medicine and Therapeutics at the University of Aberdeen and Honorary Consultant Physician/Nephrologist to the Grampian Health Board. His current interest in transplant immunology was stimulated as a Harkness Fellow at Harvard Medical School and the Peter Bent Brighton Hospital, Boston, USA. He is a member of many medical societies including the Association of Physicians of Great Britain and Ireland, the Renal Association and the Transplantation Society. He has published widely on transplant and reproductive immunology, calcium metabolism and general nephrology.

1

THE KIDNEY IN DIABETES MELLITUS

J. J. BENDING and H. KEEN

INTRODUCTION

The kidney and urinary tract in diabetes mellitus is especially prone to a number of acute complications, such as the increased frequency of urinary tract infection, the occurrence of renal papillary necrosis (a serious but perhaps diminishingly common event) and the development of the diabetic neuropathic bladder. By far the most serious chronic complication, however, is the appearance of persistent clinical proteinuria due to the development of diabetic nephropathy or intercapillary glomerulosclerosis, a major long-term sequel of the disease which has serious implications with respect to both health and lifespan in patients with insulin-dependent diabetes mellitus (IDDM) and non-insulin-dependent diabetes mellitus (NIDDM) alike.

Because of its dominating importance, this chapter will be devoted to discussion of the recent advances in knowledge concerning the epidemiology and natural history of diabetic nephropathy, newer methods for screening for this complication, and the clinical approaches which are developing as strategies in attempts to influence the natural history of the progression of diabetic nephropathy, from its first manifestations through its silent mid-term development to end-stage renal failure.

EPIDEMIOLOGY OF DIABETIC NEPHROPATHY

Diabetic nephropathy, potentially, is the single largest cause of death in patients with insulin-dependent diabetes at least in the western world. 'Potentially' because increasing numbers of diabetic patients in end-stage renal failure are now accepted on to renal support programmes, their lives extended by dialysis and transplantation; 'potentially' also because of the greatly increased risk of coronary disease and cardiovascular mortality in the proteinuric nephropathic diabetic. Epidemiological review of nephropathy prevalence in the United Kingdom presents a similar picture to that recorded in both Scandinavia and North America: approximately 30% of all patients with insulin-dependent diabetes will develop clinical proteinuria, a virtually certain indicator of advanced and progressive diabetic kidney disease after approximately 20 years. Clinical proteinuria in IDDM patients is a risk factor, not only for the progression to end-stage renal failure (ESRF), but also, as noted above, for coronary heart disease (CHD). In one ten-year follow-up of several hundred IDDM patients, 43% of those with proteinuria had died, three quarters from uraemia and one quarter from vascular causes, especially myocardial infarction, compared with only 2% of those without proteinuria. The increased risk of cardiovascular disease associated with clinical proteinuria in diabetes is probably in part due to co-existent hypertension and hyperlipidaemia which accompany diabetic nephropathy. Part of the risk of arterial disease, however, remains unexplained and may be due to increased arterial wall permeability. This could also explain the increased liability to CHD of NIDDM patients with microalbuminuria (see below).

The incidence of diabetic nephropathy in patients with NIDDM has so far been less clearly ascertained. Persistent proteinuria progressing to renal failure certainly occurs in this type of diabetes but several studies now indicate that death in such patients is more likely to be due to coronary, cerebral and generalized arterial disease. This apparently lower risk of kidney disease may simply signify that patients with late-onset diabetes pass more slowly through the phases of lesser degrees of renal impairment before progression to end-stage renal disease and the need for renal support therapy. They are, therefore, exposed longer to the atherogenic factors associated with diabetic nephropathy and so more likely to meet a cardiovascular fate. Despite this slower progression and pre-emptive mortality from arterial disease, a substantial proportion of non-insulin-dependent diabetics will nevertheless progress to ESRF and be considered for dialysis or transplantation. Although the individual risk of renal failure is relatively smaller, the prevalence of non-insulin-dependent diabetes is about four or five times that of insulin-dependent diabetes. As a consequence, the absolute numbers of non-insulin dependent diabetic patients presenting for renal support is similar to the number with insulin-dependent diabetes. In some countries and ethnic groups where NIDDM is more common and starts earlier in life, the numbers of NIDDM patients seeking renal support greatly exceed those with IDDM.

Ethnic variability in the frequency of diabetic nephropathy has been increasingly appreciated in the past few years. Diabetic patients from the Indian subcontinent, for example, have a high incidence of uraemia. Among Pima Indian, Mexican and Japanese diabetics, renal failure associated with NIDDM, is considerably more common than that associated with IDDM.

A possible explanation for the high rate of nephropathy in these NIDDM populations is that non-insulin-dependent diabetes appears earlier in life, so increasing the period of exposure to the diabetic state. Furthermore, these populations in general are at much lower risk of premature death from ischaemic heart disease.

NATURAL HISTORY OF DIABETIC NEPHROPATHY

It has been customary to date the onset of clinical nephropathy in diabetic patients from the first appearance of clinical proteinuria (exceeding 500 mg protein excreted per 24 hours) in otherwise asymptomatic patients with no history of kidney disease and with normal renal function. The phenomenon of clinical proteinuria, often defined by a positive test to the semiquantative Albustix testing strip or by a definite precipitate with sulphosalicylic acid, may appear intermittently at first (intermittent proteinuria). Even after the development of persistent clinical proteinuria there follows a 'latent' period (with a mean duration of about 5 to 7 years) of increasing proteinuria and deteriorating glomerular function during which the patient remains largely asymptomatic. The deterioration in glomerular filtration rate (GFR) is approximately linear for a given patient, although the slope of decline may vary as much as five-fold between patients. As GFR declines, arterial pressure rises and the degree of proteinuria increases.

Association with some degree of diabetic retinopathy (and often with the more severe forms of sight-threatening proliferative retinopathy and maculopathy) is almost invariable. Absence of retinopathy should raise doubts as to the cause of the proteinuria and is an indication for renal biopsy. Other specific long-term diabetic complications (such as peripheral and autonomic neuropathy) and macrovascular complications (accelerated atherosclerosis leading to coronary, peripheral vascular and cerebrovascular disease) often also co-exist.

It is this combination of pathology which has often, in the past, deterred nephrologists from taking diabetics with end-stage renal failure on to renal replacement programmes. Serum creatinine concentration does not rise above the upper range of normal until glomerular filtration rate has decreased by more than 50%. As renal failure advances, the serum creatinine rises exponentially and, if expressed as the reciprocal (l/cr), the fall in the value so obtained becomes linear with time.

The patient with chronic renal failure due to diabetic nephropathy often does not become symptomatic (with increasing fatiguability and eventual nausea and vomiting) until ESRF approaches, usually when the glomerular filtration rate has fallen below a level of $20\,\mathrm{ml\,min^{-1}\,(1.73\,m^2)^{-1}}$, and often below $10\,\mathrm{ml\,min^{-1}\,(1.73\,m^2)^{-1}}$, with a serum creatinine concentration of $600\,\mu\mathrm{mol\,L^{-1}}$ or more.

SCREENING FOR DIABETIC NEPHROPATHY

Although present strategies for intervention may sometimes be capable of slowing and perhaps even, in some cases, almost halting the decline in renal function, there is no measure which reverses the decrease. The renal lesions which are present at first appearance of clinical proteinuria are very likely to be irreversible and, in many cases, therapy appears to have little influence on the inexorable decline of renal function. This is increasing reason to suppose that if intervention is to be successful, it should be applied at an earlier stage. This fact has underlined the need for markers or predictors which will distinguish the 30% or so of IDDM patients who are at risk of developing of renal failure. Measures of prevention and intervention may then be aimed specifically at this important sub-group.

Histology and structure – function studies

In 1936, Kimmelstiel and Wilson described 'hyaline' nodules in the glomeruli of 8 elderly diabetic patients with proteinuria and/or the nephrotic syndrome. Although, for a time, it was assumed that these 'Kimmelstiel–Wilson nodules' were pathognomonic of diabetic nephropathy, it is now appreciated that they are relatively uncommon among diabetics. In one consecutive series of 200 autopsies on diabetic patients, a quarter of the patients had at least one nodule, but, even in those individuals, nodules were present in only 9% of glomeruli. The much more common histological picture seen in diabetic nephropathy is of diffuse glomerulosclerosis. A constant finding in diabetic nephropathy is the presence of glomerular basement membrane thickening, accompanied by expansion of the glomerular mesangium primarily due to the enlargement of the mesangial matrix with material which has the same properties as, and is contiguous with, the glomerular capillary basement membrane. It has been argued that the thickening of the glomerular basement membrane and, more particularly, the accumulation of the basement membrane-like material within the mesangial region, leads to mesangial expansion which progressively encroaches on the subendothelial space. This increasingly compromises and restricts the glomerular capillary lumen, reducing glomerular blood flow and leading ultimately to glomerular occlusion and sclerosis. There is a relationship between the number of glomeruli with occluded capillaries, the duration of diabetes and degree of renal failure. In other respects, however, the link between histological appearance and the degree of renal dysfunction is not close. A renal biopsy may show light microscopical changes in diabetic patients with ESRF apparently identical to abnormalities in nonproteinuric diabetics. Biopsy appearances are therefore of little value in the staging or the assessment of severity of the disease.

Hyperfiltration and nephromegaly

The phenomenon of glomerular hyperfiltration (an abnormally raised glomerular filtration rate) is found in approximately 20–30% of insulin-dependent diabetic patients of some years' standing. It has been shown to be mediated, at least in part, by raised levels of blood glucose, by some disturbed metabolites and by hormonal changes. The characteristics of this glomerular hyperfunction have been explored using micropuncture techniques in experimental diabetic rats in which the phenomenon of hyperfiltration can be predictably reproduced. It has been shown to consist mainly of profound renal vasodilatation, more marked at the afferent than the efferent glomerular arterioles, thus resulting in both increased glomerular plasma flow rate and a raised mean transglomerular hydraulic pressure gradient. The elevated GFR in humans is strongly associated with increased kidney volume (nephromegaly) which may amount to more than 60% increase in volume. A high GFR is unlikely to occur in normal-sized kidneys although a large kidney can be associated with a normal GFR. Histology of the large kidneys reveals hyperplasia and hypertrophy of the renal tubules, but only hypertrophy of the glomeruli. Glomerular hypertrophy increases the surface area available for filtration. A strong correlation has been demonstrated between GFR and the estimated glomerular filtering surface area in diabetic patients.

The exact relationship between GFR and urinary albumin excretion rate (AER) in diabetic patients without clinical proteinuria remains unresolved and awaits description in detail. In cross-sectional studies of groups of patients with diabetes of differing duration, an elevated GFR can be associated with either normal or subclinically elevated levels of albumin excretion (microalbuminuria). Microalbuminuria may, however, be accompanied by a high or normal GFR. Whether an increase in GFR precedes a rise in AER is uncertain and requires longitudinal studies of groups of patients from the time of onset of IDDM. In experimental diabetic animals, an elevated GFR has been implicated in the initiation and progression of diabetic renal disease, but this has yet to be demonstrated in humans. In one study, a small selected group of diabetic patients with hyperfiltration (several of whom also had microalbuminuria) progressed to persistent clinical proteinuria and reduced glomerular function over a ten-year period at a significantly higher rate than a control group, starting with low GFR and normal albumin excretion rate. Unfortunately, therefore, this study is unable to distinguish between hyperfiltration and microalbuminuria as the precursor of glomerular damage and loss of glomerular function, and it remains possible that hyperfiltration may play a role, perhaps independently of microalbuminuria, in diabetic glomerulosclerosis and renal failure. Whether the nephromegaly has independent predictive significance for nephropathy and whether it precedes, follows or accompanies glomerular hyperfiltration is unknown.

Microalbuminuria

The definition of proteinuria as normal or pathological has depended to some extent on the sensitivity of the detection methods used. Protein may be excreted at ten to twenty times the normal rate and yet remain below the usual clinical levels of detection. Sensitive immunoassays to measure low concentrations of albumin in the urine have shown that the albumin excretion rate in healthy individuals ranges between 2.5 and 25 mg/24 h with a geometric mean of about 9.5 mg/24 h. Diabetic patients with urine positive to Albustix testing generally have albumin excretion rates in excess of 250 mg/24 h. The wide supranormal yet subclinical range falling between 25 and 250 mg/24 h represents the rates of excretion defined for our purposes as microalbuminuria. Despite some different values attached to that term, we propose that it should be defined as the range between the upper limits of normal and the excretion rates associated with the first definite positive response of the clinical tests (e.g. Albustix) for proteinuria.

The phenomenon of microalbuminuria (as defined as above) occurs in approximately 25–30% of insulin-dependent diabetic patients. In an early prospective study of a cohort of insulin-dependent diabetics, it was found that approximately 80% of non-clinically proteinuric patients with an overnight albumin excretion rate in excess of

30 μg/min developed persistent proteinuria or were in renal failure by the time of follow up 14 years later. In contrast, only 4% of those IDDM patients with an albumin excretion rate below 30 μg/min became persistently proteinuric over the same time span. These findings, suggesting the strong predictive power of microalbuminuria, have since been supported by two other independent groups using somewhat different conditions of urine collection and definitions of microalbuminuria. The findings suggest that IDDM patients with microalbuminuria have a 20-fold higher risk of developing clinical nephropathy than patients with normal albumin excretion rates. The microalbuminuria of early diabetes appears to be glomerular in origin; tubular function as judged by urinary excretion of β_2 microglobulin is normal. In patients with microalbuminuria, the albumin excretion rate increases by an average of approximately 25% per year.

Microalbuminuria was, thus, a powerful predictor of the later development of clinical nephropathy. It remains to be determined whether the subclinically raised AER was a marker of glomerular susceptibility, distinguishing from the whole IDDM population the 30% or so who would ultimately develop diabetic renal disease, or whether it simply represented the earliest manifestation of the nephropathic process itself. The latter interpretation now seems the more likely. If microalbuminuria were a marker, one would expect to find it at (or even before) the clinical onset of IDDM. However, our recent findings indicate that levels of AER identifying at-risk patients are not found during the first five years of diabetes in conventionally treated IDDM patients. Furthermore, so far as the limited biopsy data can be interpreted, glomerular morphology in microalbuminuric patients is already markedly abnormal with thickened capillary basement membranes and mesangial expansion.

Microalbuminuria has been shown in several studies to be associated with poor glycaemic control and to be reduced (or its rate of increase slowed) by the intensification of diabetic control. An important feature of the microalbuminuric state in IDDM patients is its association with elevated levels of arterial pressure. Systolic and diastolic blood pressures are significantly higher in patients with microalbuminuria than in those matched patients with albumin excretion rates within the normal range – despite the fact that the majority of patients with microalbuminuria have arterial pressures within the normal range.

This significant increase in arterial pressure is to be found before the stage of clinical nephropathy and in the absence of renal impairment; glomerular filtration rate is either normal or elevated at this stage. This raises the question of the nature of the relationship. Are the higher blood pressures the result of early kidney pathology or does microalbuminuria occur in diabetic subjects with 'naturally' higher pressures? Or is some third factor responsible for both the elevated pressure and the susceptibility to nephropathy. If the raised pressure is not a consequence of the renal disease but a cause of it, perhaps even these early minor elevations of blood pressure should be treated with hypotensive agents. There is good evidence that effective anti-hypertensive treatment slows the rate of decrease in renal function. It is possible that effective early treatment could slow (or even stop) progression to clinical nephropathy. Several studies suggest that, over the relatively short term, treatment of microalbuminuria with anti-hypertensive drugs (e.g. angiotensin converting enzyme inhibitors; beta-blocking agents) reduces the albumin excretion rate, but longer-term studies with 'harder' end points are needed.

The search for genetic markers of susceptibility to diabetic nephropathy

The finding of raised arterial pressure early in microalbuminuric diabetics who ultimately develop diabetic nephropathy has led to recent studies demonstrating that the non-diabetic parents of IDDM patients with nephropathy have higher blood pressures than the parents of matched non-nephropathic diabetics. The hypothesis has therefore been proposed that it is those IDDM patients with an inherited predisposition to raised arterial pressure who are susceptible to nephropathy.

One of the markers of essential hypertension in non-diabetic subjects is increased activity of the red blood cell membrane sodium–lithium countertransport which represents the sodium–hydrogen exchanger in renal tubular epithelium. Sodium–lithium countertransport activity has been examined as a cell marker in normotensive offspring of hypertensive parents and found to be abnormal by some (but not all) authors. Changes in countertransport rates may not obtain in young children and in non-white races. In white adult populations, however, a growing body of evidence suggests that countertransport activity is associated with the risk of essential hypertension, aggregates in families and has a strong genetic component.

We have recently investigated the activity of the sodium–lithium countertransport system in white European adult insulin-dependent diabetic patients with nephropathy (15 patients), in insulin-dependent diabetics without nephropathy (15 patients) and in non-diabetic patients with other renal disease (15 patients). Measures of metabolic control and plasma-free insulin and growth hormone concentrations were similar in the two diabetic groups. The degree of renal functional impairment was comparable in the diabetics and non-diabetics with renal disease. Body mass index and plasma potassium concentration was similar in all three groups. Diastolic blood pressures were elevated to a similar degree in the two renal disease groups which were both above the mean pressure of the diabetics without renal disease.

Red blood cell sodium–lithium countertransport rates were found to be significantly higher in the diabetics with renal disease (0.55 ± 0.19 Li^+ mmol $(1\ RBC)^{-1}\ h^{-1}$) than in both the group of diabetics without renal disease (0.33 ± 0.16 Li^+ mmol $(1\ RBC)^{-1}\ h^{-1}$, $p < 0.005$) and in the group of non-diabetics with renal disease (0.31 ± 0.14 Li^+ mmol $(1\ RBC)^{-1}\ h^{-1}$; $p < 0.001$).

This demonstration of increased activity of red cell sodium–lithium countertransport, a marker of risk for essential hypertension, in insulin-dependent diabetics selected for nephropathy is supported by the findings of a group working separately in the USA who have made similar observations in the parents of microalbuminuric IDDM patients. These observations suggest that the hypertension of diabetic nephropathy may indeed be, not simply a secondary consequence of the renal disease, but rather an important contributor to it. This interpretation is supported by two observations:

(a) Elevated sodium–lithium countertransport rates in microalbuminuric insulin-dependent diabetics, who are, as already discussed, a group at risk of developing nephropathy but who have only a slight elevation in blood pressure without renal functional impairment, and
(b) Our data and that of others indicating that non-diabetic renal

failure with secondary hypertension is associated with normal average rates of sodium–lithium countertransport.

The mechanism by which this membrane transport disturbance could be involved in the aetiology of diabetic nephropathy in a proportion of diabetic patients remains open to speculation. Some experimental evidence supports the suggestion that the increased activity of the red cell sodium–lithium countertransport may reflect an increased activity of the renal tubule brush-border sodium–hydrogen exchanger. If this is so, it could explain the finding of enhanced sodium retention in diabetics. Those individuals who, in order to maintain sodium balance, increase systemic and renal perfusion pressure may, if they chance also to be diabetic, be the group at special risk of developing nephropathy. In the renal vasodilatory setting of diabetes, raised systemic arterial pressure would be transmitted to the glomerular microcirculation with potentially damaging effects. It is of note that the combination of arterial hypertension and diabetes leads to the most severe renal histological lesions, both in the experimental animal model and in man. Family studies in patients with diabetic nephropathy and follow-up studies of non-nephropathic diabetics with increased sodium–lithium countertransport rates are now required to confirm the genetic and predictive features of this observation.

STRATEGIES FOR INTERVENTION IN DIABETIC NEPHROPATHY

Glycaemic control

In the light of much early evidence to implicate a central role of hyperglycaemia in the genesis and progression of diabetic renal disease, as in other tissue complications associated with the diabetic state, it was natural that much early attention should be paid to the influence of intensified diabetic control on the rate of deterioration of renal function in diabetic patients with clinical nephropathy. Such studies became possible with the development of such strategies as continuous subcutaneous insulin infusion (CSII) as a tool for achieving long-term near-normoglycaemia. Estimates of efficacy of diabetic control were greatly assisted by the measurement of glycated haemoglobin as an objective integrated index of average glycaemia over the preceding two or three months. In rats with experimentally induced diabetes, strict control of glycaemia with insulin has been shown to improve morphological, histological and hyperfunction renal changes which occur in poorly controlled animals. In man, there is evidence that certain of the early changes associated with IDDM can be influenced by intensified diabetic treatment, although this did not appear to influence subsequent renal disease with detectable proteinuria.

An initial study from our group examined the effect of long-term correction of hyperglycaemia on the rate of deterioration of renal function in six insulin-dependent diabetic patients with persistent Albustix-positive proteinuria due to diabetic nephropathy. After a planned run-in observation period of 10 to 24 months to establish the individual rates of decline of function, patients entered a programme of CSII for up to 4 years. Significant and substantial long-term improvement of glycaemic control appeared to have little impact on the progression of established renal failure, glomerular filtration rate continuing to fall, plasma creatinine to rise, and fractional clearance of albumin to increase. Although no significant effect was demonstrated in the group as a whole, the number of patients was small and the possibility of heterogeneous renal responses to metabolic correction in different patients could not be excluded. Although glycaemic control during the experimental CSII period was clearly improved, as judged by several objective measures, the possibility remains that the improvement achieved still fell short of that required. There are inherent difficulties of glycaemic control in insulin-dependent diabetes which develop as nephropathy advances and which we and others have explored in some detail. Increased susceptibility to hypoglycaemia, loss of early warning symptoms and impaired recovery mechanisms conspire to induce the patient to relax over-tight control for fear of its consequences.

The failure of improved glycaemic control to influence progression when the patients had detectable proteinuria and a reduced GFR suggests that, by the time renal function is deteriorating, the nephropathic process is worsening independently of the metabolic disturbance. It has been argued that adaptive hyperfiltration in surviving nephrons, in response to the loss of others, may ultimately be self-destructive.

We, therefore, undertook a further detailed prospective study of intensified diabetic control in insulin-dependent diabetic patients with intermittent clinical proteinuria, a stage preceding the development of persistent clinical proteinuria. Even in this earlier clinical phase of diabetic nephropathy, improved glycaemic control failed to influence significantly the progression of the disease process. Although levels of GFR were still within the normal range in these intermittently proteinuric patients, the progressive rate of fall in GFR (0.9 ml min^{-1} $month^{-1}$) was comparable in magnitude with that observed during the later stages of diabetic renal failure. The rate of decline of GFR did not differ between the experimental group, randomly allocated after 12 months study to intensive insulin therapy with CSII (and significantly improved glycaemic control), and the control group who continued with their conventional insulin therapy unchanged. These studies emphasize the likelihood of a progressive pathological process established from early phases of renal involvement, even before the considerable renal functional reserve nears exhaustion and GFR starts to fall.

Studies of intensive insulin therapy at an even earlier stage of diabetic nephropathy (i.e. the stage of microalbuminuria) have been more promising. Short-term studies in Albustix-negative insulin-dependent diabetic subjects with microalbuminuria had shown that treatment with CSII significantly reduced the albumin excretion rate (AER) in a small group of microalbuminuric IDDM patients over a period of a few days. The prospective controlled eight-month Kroc Collaborative Study examined the effects of more protracted out-patient CSII-induced metabolic correction upon microalbuminuria. Twenty-four-hour urine collections obtained at baseline, at four and eight months of the trial, were available from 59 Albustix-negative patients. β_2-Microglobulin (a marker of tubular function) was normal. The 39 normoalbuminuric patients (AER, $<12\,\mu g/min$) did not differ significantly from the 20 patients in whom AER was elevated above our upper limits of normal and lay between 13.2 and 192.6 $\mu g/min$ with respect to distributions of age, sex and duration of diabetes. In both the normoalbuminuric group and the group with elevated excretion rates studied at 4 and 8 months, %HbA_1 and mean blood glucose were significantly decreased during CSII compared with baseline values, whereas no change occurred in the group continuing their conventional insulin therapy (CIT).

AER did not differ between CIT and CSII treatment groups in the normoalbuminuric patients. However, AER fell significantly in the CSII-treated patients with elevated excretion rates at 4 and 8 months ($p<0.01$) but showed no significant change in the patients with supranormal AER in the CIT group. In patients with a known high risk of progression to clinical nephropathy (i.e. those with AER > 30 μg/min), four out of four improved during CSII, but only two out of six during CIT. These results, therefore, strongly suggest a significant and sustained reduction of abnormally raised rates of urinary albumin excretion in IDDM patients. Other groups have subsequently found a tendency of strict glycaemic control to slow or halt the rise in AER in microalbuminuric IDDM patients over longer periods of time.

Arterial pressure control

In patients with established diabetic nephropathy, blood pressure rises as the GFR declines. However, as already discussed, significantly elevated levels of arterial pressure occur in the stage of microalbuminuria when glomerular function is preserved. With the appearance of persistent proteinuria, linear decline of GFR is inexorably established and has usually fallen to clearly abnormally low levels 5–10 years later. The rate of decline varies in different individuals, ranging from 0.5–2.5 ml min^{-1} $month^{-1}$, but the factors determining the different speeds of fall are little known. It has been suggested that one such determinant is the level of arterial pressure although this has not been confirmed by others. There is no doubt however that effective blood pressure treatment is valuable in conserving renal function and has been estimated to slow the rate of decline of GFR by an average of 5–6 ml min^{-1} $year^{-1}$. In a small but carefully followed series, vigorous treatment of raised blood pressure in patients with persistent clinical proteinuria lowered the rate of decline of GFR from 0.9 ml min^{-1} $month^{-1}$ before treatment to 0.24 ml min^{-1} $month^{-1}$ during treatment. This lower rate of fall was maintained for several years. Concomitantly, the degree of proteinuria was significantly reduced, though it remained within the clinically positive range.

This slowing of the rate of decline in renal function by effective blood pressure control was obtained in the absence of special efforts to intensify blood glucose control or alter dietary habits. The antihypertensive regimens used in these early studies included selective β-adrenergic blocking agents, vasodilators and diuretics. More recently, a number of studies, mostly uncontrolled and small in size, suggest that the administration of angiotensin converting enzyme (ACE) inhibitors to diabetic patients in renal failure may have an additional specific beneficial effect on the progression of renal disease. Some workers have suggested that this improvement is independent of systemic blood pressure reduction. Animal studies indicate that the amelioration of the nephropathic process may be related to the lowering of intraglomerular pressure. Most evidence thus supports the view that, by the time declining GFR is demonstrable, the process leading to end-stage renal failure has become independent of the metabolic disturbance of diabetes. In this phase, haemodynamic factors in established nephropathy have become predominant determinants of progression of renal damage.

Dietary protein restriction

Dietary protein has been implicated for some years in the progression of glomerular failure in chronic renal failure. There is evidence in animals and man that the levels of dietary protein ingested by Western man are associated with an increase in GFR, increased renal blood flow and intrarenal hypertension – haemodynamic changes that under pathological conditions, such as those occurring in diabetes, may be important in the genesis of progressive glomerular damage. Dietary protein restriction has been used for decades to alleviate the symptoms of end-stage renal failure. The use of less rigid low-protein diets in earlier stages of chronic renal failure of various causes has more recently been shown to delay the progression to end-stage disease and the need for renal support therapy. The long-term effect of dietary protein on the progression of diabetic nephropathy in this phase had not been studied systematically, however, and the practical possibility of this approach has been questioned.

Over the past few years at Guys Hospital, we have been studying the effect of restricting dietary protein intake to 40 g/day in a fairly large cohort of insulin-dependent diabetic patients. They have been submitted to frequent detailed clinical and laboratory assessments of renal function, including urinary protein excretion studies and measurements of GFR (using the ^{51}Cr EDTA clearance technique). Twenty-one patients studied had persistent clinical proteinuria due to diabetic nephropathy. GFRs ranged from severely impaired renal function to those still in the normal range. Patients were studied while taking their usual protein diets for 48 months, in order to establish baseline rates of renal decline, and then for 28 months after the prescription of a low-protein diet (40 g/day). Patients were thus used as their own controls, in a situation in which decline in renal function is largely linear for a given patient.

Achieved long-term dietary protein intake fell to 46 g protein/day from a previous mean of 84 g protein/day. A small initial fall in body weight did not continue and mid-arm muscle circumference did not change. Reduction in dietary protein intake (confirmed by a fall in urinary urea excretion in addition to dietary history) was accompanied by a fall in circulating plasma urea concentration and total urinary protein excretion (which would have been expected to continue to rise). The effect on GFR was to slow the rate of decline from a group mean of 0.7 ml min^{-1} $month^{-1}$ to 0.14 ml min^{-1} $month^{-1}$. There were no sequential changes in HbA_1 levels or supine mean blood pressure.

Thus, it appears that, at least in our study, the prescription of a moderate dietary protein restriction (which proved acceptable to most patients in the long term) may significantly slow the decline to end-stage renal disease, and should be particularly considered at an early stage of the disease. The involvement of a dedicated dietician is essential, but the patients themselves are generally very motivated to accept what is a matter of great importance to their prognosis. The application of dietary protein restriction (in addition to the careful control of blood pressure and perhaps having additive beneficial effects) may allow some years or more of asymptomatic adequate renal function in those patients who are likely to develop end-stage renal failure and may ultimately require dialysis and/or transplantation.

FURTHER READING

1. Andersen, A. R., Christiansen, J. S., Andersen, J. K., Kreiner, S. and Deckert, T. (1983). Diabetic nephropathy in Type 1 (insulin-dependent) diabetes: an epidemiological study. *Diabetologia*, **25,** 496–501
2. Viberti, G. C. and Keen, H. (1984). The patterns of proteinuria in diabetes mellitus. Relevance to pathogenesis and prevention of diabetic nephropathy. *Diabetes*, **33,** 686–692
3. Bending, J. J., Viberti, G. C., Watkins, P. J. and Keen, H. (1986). Intermittent clinical proteinuria and renal function in diabetes: evolution and the effect of glycaemic control. *Br. Med. J.*, **292,** 83–96
4. Viberti, G. C., Wiseman, M. J. and Bending, J. J. (1986). Prevention of diabetic nephropathy: markers of disease and perspectives for intervention. *Diabetic Med.*, **3,** 208–211
5. Bending, J. J., Pickup, J. C., Viberti, G. C. and Keen, H. (1984). Glycaemic control in diabetic nephropathy. *Br. Med. J.*, **288,** 487–491
6. Mangili, R., Bending, J. J., Scott, G., Li, L. K., Gupta, A. and Viberti, G. C. (1988). Increased sodium–lithium countertransport activity in red cells of patients with insulin-dependent diabetes and nephropathy. *N. Engl. J. Med.*, **318,** 146–150

2

MULTIPLE MYELOMA AND RENAL FUNCTION

S. M. CRAWFORD

HISTORICAL INTRODUCTION

Thomas Alexander McBean died on New Year's Day, 1846, the cause of his death being certified as atrophy from albuminuria. Clamp[1] has identified this man as being the source of the specimen of urine which Dr Thomas Watson sent to Dr Henry Bence Jones on 1st November, 1845. This urine contained a substance which Bence Jones characterized according to the understanding of chemistry in the mid-nineteenth century[2] and which we now know as Bence Jones protein.

The clinical features presented by Mr McBean were summarized by Bence Jones[3].

> 'When I saw the patient, there was excessive emaciation; yellowish skin, clear conjunctivae, lips dry, tongue fissured, moist, furred at the back, pulse 85, small, skin moist, bowels – tendency to diarrhoea, motions reported not unhealthy, urine not passed in large quantities, no urgency – no frequency, pinkish urates deposited, much mucous râles in the chest, over-strong pulsation of the heart, complained of pain in the left shoulder and side, was obliged to be moved most gently in bed on account of the pain.'

Six weeks after Bence Jones saw him the patient died. At necropsy, the remarkable feature was the softness of the bones which gave rise to the original name given to the condition: Mollities ossium[4,5].

Over the next 100 years, this disease became better understood as a clinical syndrome characterized by pain associated with multiple osteolytic lesions. Serum proteins were commonly elevated, with Bence Jones proteinuria being detected by the classical heat test in over half the patients. Renal dysfunction occurred in 60% of patients according to the series reported by Bayrd and Heck[6].

MULTIPLE MYELOMA AND LYMPHOID NEOPLASIA

We now know that this disease consists of a malignant proliferation of plasma cells. Since these cells present the end stage of the differentiation process in the B cell lymphocytic line, myeloma bears a relationship with the other neoplasms of this group of cells[7] so that, for example, monoclonal free immunoglobulin light chains may be found in the urine of patients with lymphoma[8].

Monoclonal proliferations of B lymphocytes may, like other tumours, be benign or malignant. When the cells concerned are plasma cells, they frequently produce an immunoglobulin in an amount exceeding the production of protein by other clones of similar cells. Since the protein molecules produced by individual cells within a clone all have an identical primary structure, they are electrophoretically homogeneous, producing the characteristic M-spike on electrophoresis of the patient's serum. When this is detected, the clinician has to decide whether this monoclonal gammopathy is benign or malignant.

The features which help to differentiate benign from malignant monoclonal gammopathy have been described in the clinical study by Hobbs[9]. Some patients have a malignant condition other than multiple myeloma, such as non-Hodgkin lymphoma, Waldenstrom's macroglobulinaemia or chronic lymphocytic leukaemia. In that study, a diagnosis of multiple myeloma was accepted if, in addition to paraproteinaemia, there was evidence of bone involvement (either discrete osteolytic lesions or diffuse bone loss with pathological fractures) or histological evidence of an excess of atypical plasma cells. In patients who did not entirely fulfil the above criteria, the features which were associated with a rapid increase in the level of the paraprotein during observation, and therefore a firm diagnosis of myeloma, were Bence Jones proteinuria and reduced levels of other immunoglobulins. In addition, those patients who had a serum paraprotein concentration greater than 10 g/L tended to have a malignant clone. Those who did, usually exhibited one of the above features. The presence of Bence Jones protein or immunosuppression was not in itself a criterion of malignancy – indeed, Bence Jones gammopathy may follow a benign course[10]. Tubbs *et al.*[11] have described eleven patients who had renal failure due to light chain deposition; in only four of them was a confident diagnosis of multiple myeloma made.

Kyle[12], reporting his observations of 241 patients with monoclonal gammopathy of undetermined significance, found that 27 (11 per cent) went on to develop frank multiple myeloma. The median interval before this diagnosis was established was 64 months (range 23 to 136). This author has described seven patients with idiopathic Bence Jones proteinuria who have been followed up for a long period[13]. Five of these patients went on to develop multiple myeloma.

DIAGNOSTIC CRITERIA

Treatment decisions in plasma cell neoplasia depend on defined criteria by which to assign patients to the benign or malignant classification. The most precise are those of the South West Oncology Group of the USA (Table 2.1)[14]. In addition to these formal criteria, the diagnosis may be supported by non-specific features, namely anaemia, hypercalcaemia, uraemia, osteoporosis with compression fractures and hypoalbuminaemia. These criteria are more complex than the standard criteria[15] employed by the UK Medical Research Council (MRC), which are the presence of a paraprotein spike, osteolytic lesion, and bone marrow infiltration with plasma cells. A patient is considered to have multiple myeloma by these criteria if at least two are fulfilled. The difficulty with regard to these criteria is the disagreement between haematologists regarding what constitutes marrow infiltration and the possibility that another condition may be responsible for any marrow plasmacytosis[15]. This question is discussed by Parker and Malpas[16].

TABLE 2.1 Criteria for diagnosis of multiple myeloma[14]

MAJOR CRITERIA

I. Plasmacytomas on tissue biopsy
II. Bone marrow plasmacytosis (>30% plasma cells)
III. Monoclonal globulin spike: >35 g/L (IgG) >20 g/L (IgA) or kappa or lambda chain excretion >1.0 g/day

MINOR CRITERIA

a. Bone marrow plasmacytosis (10–30%)
b. Monoclonal globulin spike present, but less than levels defined in III above
c. Lytic bone lesions
d. Polyclonal immunoglobulins reduced (IgM<0.5 g/L, IgA<1 g/L, IgG<6 g/L)

In symptomatic patients, the following features or combination of features confirm the diagnosis:

i. I+b, c or d
ii. II+b, c or d
iii. II
iv. a+b+c; a+b+d

VARIATIONS IN PARAPROTEIN PRODUCTION

Rarely, multiple myeloma may be confirmed from radiological and histological studies but no paraprotein is detected in serum or urine. Such patients account for about 2% of those in whom multiple myeloma is diagnosed[17–19]. On the other hand, around 20% of patients have a tumour which does not produce complete immunoglobulins but only light chains[19–21]. The majority of patients have intact immunoglobulin IgG or IgA (Table 2.2). About half of all patients with myeloma have a positive heat test for Bence Jones protein although the limitations of that test are well known[22]. The urine may have to be concentrated to find this substance[9]. Radial immunodiffusion is a superior method and is quantitative[23]. Free light chains may polymerize and then be detected in serum[24]. The class of paraprotein and its chemical behaviour determine some of the clinical features of multiple myeloma[21,25–27].

TABLE 2.2 Frequency of paraprotein types

	Pruzanski et al.[21]	*West Yorkshire Series*
IgG	61%	58%
IgA	19%	25%
Light chain	20%	17%

EPIDEMIOLOGY

Multiple myeloma accounts for about 1% of cancer deaths[28] and the death rate appears to be slowly rising. This change may be due to improving diagnostic standards[29,30] or may be genuine. There is also evidence, within the British Isles, of geographical variation in the incidence of the disease[28,31]. Geographical variations have also been identified in the USA[32].

The incidence of multiple myeloma rises steeply with age, and, in most series, the mean or median age at diagnosis is between 60 and 65 (mean 62.7 in the 62 patients in the West Yorkshire series). There is higher male predominance (35 males, 27 females in the West Yorkshire series) and there is an increased incidence in black populations and a reduced incidence in oriental populations compared with European white populations[30].

Multiple myeloma seems to be associated with radiation exposure and occupational exposure to heavy metals[30].

FACTORS IN THE PROGNOSIS OF MULTIPLE MYELOMA

The best-known clinical staging system in multiple myeloma is that of Durie and Salmon[33]. The basis of this scheme is the calculation of the tumour mass borne by the patient. This was calculated by comparing *in vivo* production of the monoclonal protein characteristic of the disease with the rate of production of protein by each cell, determined *in vitro*. The tumour mass thus calculated was correlated with the clinical features observed in their reference group, and the staging

TABLE 2.3 Durie–Salmon staging system[33]

	I	*II*	*III*
No. tumour cells ($\times 10^{12}/m^2$)	<0.6	0.6–1.2	>1.2
Haemoglobin (g/dl)	>10	Fitting	<8.5
Calcium (mmol/L)	<3	neither	>3
Bone X-ray changes	Normal or solitary lesion	stage I nor	Advanced bone lesions
M component IgA (g/dl)	<30	stage III	>50
M component IgG (g/dl)	<50		>70
Bence Jones protein (g/24 h)	<4		>12

Subclassification: A serum creatinine <177 μmol/L
B serum creatinine ⩾177 μmol/L
All criteria must be fulfilled for stage I to obtain; only one of the criteria need be fulfilled to assign a patient to stage III

system in Table 2.3 was derived from these data. Whilst it has been shown independently that survival in multiple myeloma is related to tumour mass estimated in this way[34], this staging scheme has been criticized on two grounds: firstly it assigns a high proportion of patients to stage III[16] and secondly it lays little emphasis on renal involvement, which is merely a means of subclassification. It must be said, however, that it was not the intention of the authors only to provide an indication of prognosis, but to permit a continued assessment of patients in respect of tumour burden[33,35]. A further problem has been the difficulty of assessing paraprotein production, and hence tumour burden, in patients with light chain myeloma. This problem has, however, been overcome recently[36].

There have been many studies which have sought the clinical and laboratory features which indicate prognosis in myeloma patients[37–46]. Without exception, they include some measurement of glomerular function as being of great, if not supreme, prognostic importance. Other features which have been of value in this respect are haemoglobin level, Bence Jones proteinuria, performance status, serum calcium level, serum albumin, extent of bone lesions, paraprotein class and light chain type[21,47] and tritiated thymidine labelling index[43]. These clinical and other features are correlated with the degree of malignant cytological change[48,49]. The MRC analysis[38] of prognostic factors has generated a staging system based on urea, haemoglobin and

TABLE 2.4 MRC staging scheme[38]

Stage I	Urea $\leqslant$ 8 mmol/L Haemoglobulin > 10 g/dl Minimal or no symptoms
Stage II	Fitting neither I nor III
Stage III	Restricted activity AND EITHER urea > 10 mmol/L OR haemoglobulin $\geqslant$ 7.5 g/dl

performance status (Table 2.4). This has been independently assessed to be the best indicator of prognosis using standard measurements[50].

There is evidence that the serum level of β_2 microglobulin can give information regarding the state of the disease, independent of renal function, and that this can be used to assess probable survival[51–54]. Indeed, it has been shown that other commonly used indices of prognosis do not contribute any further predictive power to a statistical model over and above that of the β_2 microglobulin[55]. A subsequent study has largely confirmed this, and shown that the serum β_2 microglobulin also indicates the prognosis of patients in the plateau phase[56]. Figure 2.1 shows the use of β_2 microglobulin for stratification in myeloma. A dissenting opinion has been expressed by van Dobbenburgh *et al.*[57] who, although they confirmed that this parameter conveys prognostic information, did not find that it was superior to myeloma cell mass, serum creatinine and age. However, a single biochemical parameter that can be measured by a central laboratory has advantages as a means of stratification in a clinical trial over complex multivariate schemes.

Patients with Bence Jones myeloma (light chain disease) have a poorer prognosis than those whose tumours produce a complete immunoglobulin molecule[58,44,38]. Lambda light chain disease is said to carry a worse prognosis than kappa[27].

Amyloidosis associated with multiple myeloma has a slightly worse prognosis than when either condition occurs alone[59]. It commonly presents as carpal tunnel syndrome, but cardiac and gastrointestinal presentations are seen. When amyloid is being considered as a cause for the nephrotic syndrome, Alexanian *et al.*[59] recommended that rectal biopsy is performed before renal biopsy.

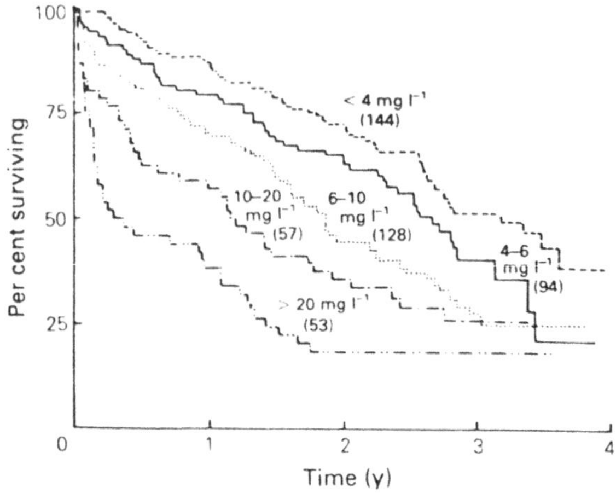

FIGURE 2.1 Survival probabilities for patients according to presentation values of serum β_2-microglobulin. Numbers in parentheses indicate numbers of patients in each group. χ^2 (trend) = 58.2; $p<0.0001$. (Reproduced with permission from *British Journal of Cancer.*)

LONG-TERM SURVIVAL

Whilst multiple myeloma is often amenable to treatment, it remains incurable. The patients who entered the first MRC myeloma trial have been followed up and the long-term results have been collated[60]. The features which have previously been referred to as indicating prognosis, e.g. renal function, haemoglobin, did not have any predictive function beyond the first five years. Acute myeloid leukaemia was the cause of death in six patients, all of whom had received continuous melphalan therapy and had been in the trial for more than four years. 45% of deaths beyond five years were due to myelomatosis, the mode of death being acute advancement of the disease or, in three of the 15 deaths due to myeloma, renal failure. Eighteen deaths which were not directly ascribed to myeloma occurred in the group of long-term survivors. Seven of these deaths were due to second malignancies, including four cases of acute myeloid leukaemia.

Alexanian[61] has investigated the characteristics of patients who survive 10 years or more and found that they were less than 65 years old at diagnosis and with low or intermediate tumour burden. They had usually responded well to chemotherapy both initially and in relapse. None presented with renal impairment or hypercalcaemia.

MANAGEMENT OF MYELOMA

Patients in whom this diagnosis is made require estimation of blood urea and creatinine, electrolytes, serum protein electrophoresis and quantification of each class of immunoglobulins and measurement of haemoglobin, white cell count and platelets. Transfusion may be indicated if the haemoglobin is less than 9 g/dl and the patient has symptoms of anaemia, but hyperviscosity should first be excluded. When the patient is dehydrated, and especially if he is hypercalcaemic, the first priority is to correct fluid and electrolyte imbalance. The blood urea should not be used as a prognostic indicator until this has been done.

Hypercalcaemia demands vigorous hydration with isotonic saline (up to 4 L per day) with potassium supplements, corticosteroids and frusemide if necessary.

Plasma viscosity should be measured in patients with clinical features of hyperviscosity (Table 2.5). Treatment for this is urgent plasmapheresis. Any infection demands vigorous treatment with broad spectrum antibiotics after appropriate specimens have been taken for culture. This is particularly important in patients who are neutropenic, either because of the degree of marrow involvement or because of chemotherapy. The regimen should include a broad spectrum β-lactam drug with antipseudomonal activity plus an aminoglycoside. Herpes virus infection can be very severe and should be managed with acyclovir[62] or other antiviral agents.

Oral candidiasis is common in patients receiving chemotherapy and should be treated with nystatin suspension or pastilles. If this drug is introduced promptly, it is often sufficient on its own, but refractory patients can be treated with amphotericin B lozenges, miconazole gel or oral ketoconazole.

A careful skeletal survey is required as a diagnostic and staging procedure and to investigate sites of bone pain. This symptom may be readily controlled by radiotherapy, but, where there is danger of pathological fracture, prophylactic internal fixation may be indicated. Neurological features suggesting spinal cord or cauda equina compression demand that a myelogram is performed.

Renal failure requires active management[63], including dialysis if necessary[64]. The MRC fourth trial specifically addressed the question

TABLE 2.5 Clinical features of hyperviscosity (associated with values >4 centipoise (4×10^3 N.S. m^{-2})

Bleeding
Purpura and bruising
Epistaxis
Mucosal bleeding
Retinopathy
Dilated retinal veins
Retinal haemorrhage
Papilloedema
Neurological symptoms
Weakness
Headache
Vertigo
Nystagmus
Limb paralysis
Coma
Hypervolaemia
Venous distension
Cardiac failure

of management of renal failure[65]. Patients who were oliguric at presentation were rehydrated and dialysed. A policy of encouraging oral fluid intake of at least 3 L/day following recovery was pursued for all patients achieving adequate urine output. This resulted in a substantial improvement in the survival of patients presenting with renal failure compared with a historical control group; half of the treated patients were alive one year after diagnosis, compared with only 20% of control patients. There was still a substantial number of deaths in the first two months of treatment.

It has been suggested that the nephrotoxicity of a light chain may be related to the isoelectric point, higher pI implying greater toxicity[66]. This observation suggests that rendering the urine alkaline might mitigate the toxic effect. The trend for patients in the 5th MRC study[65] so treated to live longer did not approach statistical significance ($p = 0.26$). The light chains from 43 of these patients were investigated for the relationship of the pI to nephrotoxicity. No relationship between light chain pI and renal failure was identified, but it was shown that tubular proteinuria (as α_1 microglobulin excretion) correlated with light chain pI[67].

Chemotherapy is indicated in patients who fulfil the criteria for diagnosis of myeloma and who are symptomatic. There is no advantage in offering chemotherapy to asymptomatic patients.

Standard chemotherapy consists of oral melphalan, which is an alkylating agent, and a glucocorticoid, usually prednisolone. The schedule used in the 4th MRC trial[68] was melphalan, 10 mg daily for 7 days, with prednisolone, 40 mg daily for 7 days, repeated every 4 weeks. Three-weekly schedules are possible, using 4–7 days treatment, titrated so as to ensure that sufficient melphalan is given to treat the tumour effectively without exposing the patient to the risk of the complications of myelosuppression[16]. However, since a 3-week schedule results in treatment falling due at the time of the haematological nadir of the previous course, resulting in delayed and missed treatments, a longer schedule may be preferable[69].

In this disease, as in others[70], it seems that response rates depend on dose intensity. Several studies have looked for means of improving chemotherapy by adding drugs to the basic alkylating and glucocorticoid regimen. No evidence of benefit was found when vincristine was added to melphalan and prednisolone[68]. The most recent MRC study compared a combination of four cytotoxic drugs (doxorubicin, BCNU, cyclophosphamide and melphalan) with melphalan, both without steroids. This study has shown a small advantage for the more complex regimen[71].

Other approaches to intense therapy include very high-dose alkylating agent chemotherapy[72]. This produces a high frequency of complete responses (27% in previously untreated patients[73]) with total abolition of the paraprotein and a normal bone marrow but patients eventually relapse and the disease is not cured.

The VAD regimen, which has attracted considerable attention recently, employs a 4-day continuous infusion of vincristine (0.4 mg/day) and doxorubicin (adriamycin 9 mg (m^2 body surface area)$^{-1}$ day^{-1}) repeated every 28 days, together with dexamethasone 40 mg/day on a 4-day-on-4-day-off cycle[74]. Response to this treatment was excellent, with 14 of 20 patients resistant to alkylating agents achieving 75% reduction in the paraprotein concentration, responses being associated with extended survival. Investigation of the VAD combination compared with dexamethasone alone has shown that the steroid is active even when patients were unresponsive to previous cytotoxic drugs, but, in patients who relapse following chemotherapy, the doxorubicin and vincristine are necessary[75].

Chemotherapy for active multiple myeloma is an essential part of patient management but it remains far from satisfactory. In order to improve understanding, it is therefore essential that every patient who presents is entered into a formal clinical trial if he meets the criteria of the protocol. As optimal use of chemotherapy involves steering a careful course between the benefits and adverse effects, experience is necessary. It is advisable that the treatment of patients requiring cytotoxic drugs should be undertaken by one team within any one institution.

Interferon-α_2 has activity in multiple myeloma[76], including those in relapse[77], but its role requires much further investigation. Double hemibody radiotherapy is a form of treatment which may have some value in difficult cases of multiple myeloma[78,79].

Progress and monitoring of patients with multiple myeloma

During his observation of a patient with myeloma, the physician has to make decisions based on predictions about how the patient's disease will fare in the immediate future. Such decisions include questions about whether chemotherapy may be stopped or whether a more aggressive regime should be instituted. Serial measurements of paraprotein levels in serum and urine[80] are principal means of monitoring on which such predictions are made. This concept has been developed to the extent that serum paraprotein levels have been used as a direct measure of changes in tumour cell mass[35]. There is a danger in this simplistic approach; during relapse, the biological nature of the tumour may change so that it produces proportionately less paraprotein, a greater proportion of Bence Jones protein, or a different paraprotein[80,81]. In assessing the initial response to therapy, however, monitoring of paraprotein levels holds pride of place.

Opinion is divided about what constitutes a response. In keeping with standard oncological practice, a partial response is frequently defined as a reduction by 50% in the paraprotein[15], implying a 50% reduction in cell mass. Others, e.g. Barlogie *et al.*[74], define partial response as >75% reduction.

It is now accepted that when paraprotein levels are stable for six months, chemotherapy is contraindicated because the evidence suggests that there is little cell turnover in the stable plateau phase[43]. This plateau is achieved by 44% of patients while a further 9% of patients enjoy a complete response[43]. It is clear that no active treatment is indicated when serum and urine paraprotein concentrations have been stable for 6 months[68,82].

It has been suspected for some time that those patients whose paraprotein levels fell quickly on treatment did less well than the others[39,40] and this belief gained further support in the 4th MRC trial[71]. There was no evidence from that study that a prolonged course of chemotherapy should be given to slow responders.

Detection of relapse depends on monitoring the patient's clinical condition and serum paraprotein levels[78]. In those patients who have tumours which produce hypercalcaemia, however, the serum calcium concentration is a very sensitive indicator of relapse and predicts the development of renal impairment[83].

RENAL LESIONS IN MULTIPLE MYELOMA

Renal failure is a feature of the early part of the course of the disease where its effect on prognosis is paramount. It has less effect in the later phase. Buckman *et al.*[60] accepted blood urea concentrations persistently raised for at least one month as their definition of renal failure. Five of the thirty-eight patients who survived five or more years died of renal failure; in one of these, the cause of the renal failure was hypertensive nephrosclerosis. This incidence of late myelomatous renal failure compares with the overall incidence of death from renal involvement of 21%[19].

Precipitation of globulins within the nephron has long been considered relevant in the development of renal lesions in myeloma[84–86]. It has become clear, however, that the kidney is affected by processes other than the simple obstruction of tubules.

Anatomical changes

Kapadia[19] has reported 62 consecutive cases of multiple myeloma which came to autopsy. He found that one-third of patients had enlarged kidneys. His histological findings are listed in Table 2.6. He found little correlation between the severity of histological changes and impairment of renal function as measured by the blood urea nitrogen except in those patients with markedly impaired function (BUN 80 mg/dl, equivalent to a blood urea concentration of 23 mmol/L).

TABLE 2.6 Histological features of the kidney in myeloma: a report of 60 autopsies[19]

FINDING	*NUMBER* (%)
Tubular atrophy and fibrosis	46 (77)
Tubular hyaline casts	37 (62)
Tubular epithelial giant cell reaction	29 (48)
Nephrocalcinosis	25 (42)
Chronic pyelonephritis	14 (23)
Acute pyelonephritis	12 (20)
Plasma cell infiltrates	6 (10)
Amyloid	3 (5)
Normal	7 (12)

More recently, Rota and colleagues[87] have found that global tubular atrophy is absent from the kidneys of patients with readily reversible renal failure. All patients had, however, some degree of epithelial degeneration or necrosis.

The classical renal lesion in multiple myeloma is termed myeloma kidney. This is defined as a lesion characterized by the presence of typical tubular casts with surrounding multinucleated cellular reactions. Cohen and Border[88] have examined renal biopsies from four patients who presented with acute renal failure. These patients had not previously been diagnosed as having multiple myeloma; indeed, the diagnosis was first made on renal biopsy evidence[89].

The dominant feature found by these authors was pronounced cast formation, principally in the distal tubules, but affecting all segments in two of their four cases. These casts had the classical fractured appearance which is associated with myeloma kidney. They were associated with tubular basement membrane damage, as well as multinucleate giant cell reaction. The tubules which did not contain casts were remarkable for what the authors describe as 'protein reabsorption droplets'. The glomeruli were largely normal, the only pathological feature being mild ischaemic changes and complete sclerosis of 10–15% of the glomerular population of each biopsy. This sparing of the glomeruli is inconsistent with the earlier electron microscopical findings of Abrahams, Pirani and Pollak[90] who demonstrated basement membrane thickening in the glomeruli.

Immunological studies demonstrated light chains of *both* classes, together with evidence of immunoglobulin heavy chains and other proteins in the tubular casts. This suggests that the casts cannot be regarded simply as precipitates of Bence Jones protein.

All these four patients, therefore, had lesions predominantly affecting renal tubules, with little damage to the glomeruli, yet all presented with an elevated serum creatinine concentration, indicating reduced glomerular filtration[89]. The renal failure of multiple myeloma, in so far as it is the consequence of myeloma kidney, is a result of renal tubular damage.

Functional changes

Tubular damage may be mild, and not associated with reduced glomerular filtration. In these circumstances, it may manifest as specific impairment of tubular function which can be detected by appropriate tests. The classical example is the adult Fanconi syndrome[91]. The features may be present long before there is clear evidence of multiple myeloma[92]. This syndrome is associated with intracellular crystalloid structures in the proximal tubules[93], although it has been described in a patient with nodular amyloid deposition which was again associated with kappa chain excretion[94].

Most reports of the Fanconi syndrome in multiple myeloma have concerned patients with a kappa-chain-producing tumour[92,93]. Rawlings *et al.*[95] have, however, reported a case involving a lambda-secreting tumour. Frank Fanconi syndrome is not the only manifestation of tubular dysfunction which may occur in this disease. De

Fronzo *et al.*[96] found defects of renal acidifying and concentrating function only in patients with Bence Jones proteinuria; only one of their 35 patients had glycosuria and aminoaciduria. At the other extreme, Smithline and colleagues[97] described a patient with Fanconi syndrome, diabetes insipidus and distal renal tubular acidosis and kappa light chain excretion in the urine, but no evidence of myeloma. Sanchez and Domz[98] also reported a patient with renal tubular acidosis; this patient had myeloma kidney with amyloidosis. Distal renal tubular acidosis is a very rare complication of myeloma[99].

Pathogenesis of renal disease

Agreement is widespread among workers in this field that Bence Jones proteinuria is the most important factor in the development of myeloma kidney[98,100–103]. Clyne *et al.*[104] have performed experiments in rats injected with large quantities of Bence Jones protein (type kappa) which produced proximal tubular abnormalities, both functional and morphological. Distal tubules were little affected. However, as Beaufils and Morel-Maroger point out[105], there is no consistent quantitive relationship between the amount of light chain excretion and the type or degree of renal dysfunction.

Cooper *et al.*[106] have studied low molecular weight proteinuria and lysosomal enzyme excretion in myeloma. Patients were found to secrete α_1 microglobulin and α_1 acid glycoprotein and, to a lesser extent, *N*-acetyl-βD-glucosaminodase if they had elevated serum creatinine. If the creatinine was normal, tubular proteinuria depended on light chain excretion. The findings support the concept that light chain toxicity to the tubule is the prime event in pathogenesis of renal disease.

Myeloma kidney occurs less commonly in IgD myeloma, although Bence Jones proteinuria type lambda is almost always present[102]. The observations of Stone and Frenkel[20] support this. This association of the Fanconi syndrome with kappa chain production has already been mentioned, and this class of light chain is associated with peritubular deposition[107,108]. In contrast, lambda chains tend to be deposited evenly both in glomerular and tubular basement membranes[11].

Kappa chains have been shown to accumulate in renal basement membranes and may be associated with the glomerular sclerosis which occurs in some patients[109]. This phenomenon has been reported in a patient who had no other evidence of paraprotein secretion[110], illustrating that the quantity of Bence Jones protein required to damage the kidney may be smaller than can at present be detected: the adult Fanconi syndrome mentioned above is another example. However, large quantities of Bence Jones protein may be excreted in some individuals without there being any impairment of renal function[111,112]. The pathogenetic role of this protein is not in doubt both from clinical and pathological studies in patients with myeloma, and from animal experiments, such as those of Koss, Pirani and Ossermann[113].

Acute renal failure

Dehydration and acute renal failure are a further manifestation of myeloma in kidney function. When dehydration follows infection[101] or is associated with intravenous urography, acute renal failure may result. De Fronzo *et al.*[114] described 14 patients who developed acute renal failure during the course of development of their myelomata. The renal histology in these patients demonstrated tubular atrophy rather than myeloma kidney. A striking feature of this group of patients was that nine of the fourteen were suffering from hypercalcaemia. The cause and effect relationship between hypercalcaemia and renal failure is complex[115]. Whilst dehydration and reduced urine output associated with acute renal failure are, in part, causes of hypercalcaemia, the calcium abnormality usually precedes the impairment of renal function[83].

The dynamic aspects of the relationship between serum calcium and renal function are illustrated in Figure 2.2.

HYPERCALCAEMIA AND RENAL FAILURE IN MYELOMA

Hypercalcaemia has a wide variety of metabolic effects[116–119]. Humes[120] has suggested that disordered calcium metabolism is the final common pathway in ischaemic and toxic acute renal failure. The effects of hypercalcaemia on the kidney were reviewed in 1968 by Epstein[121]. He

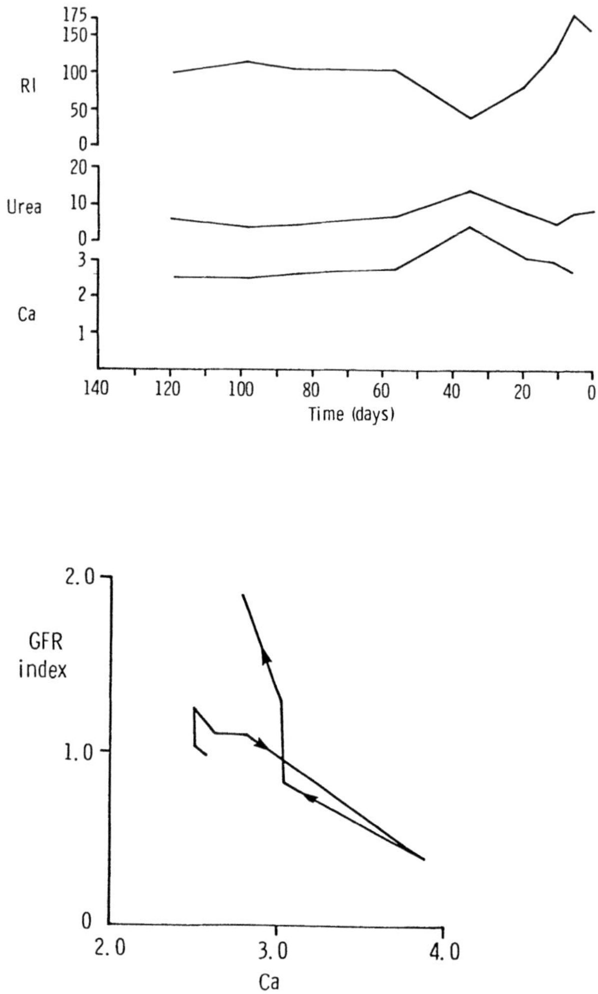

a

FIGURE 2.2 Relationship of glomular filtration rate (GFR), assessed by serum creatinine, to serum calcium concentration in patients dying from multiple myeloma associated with hypercalcaemia. (a) A patient whose GFR fell following a rise in serum calcium; treatment by hydration and steroids resulted in improved renal function but the serum calcium remained abnormal.

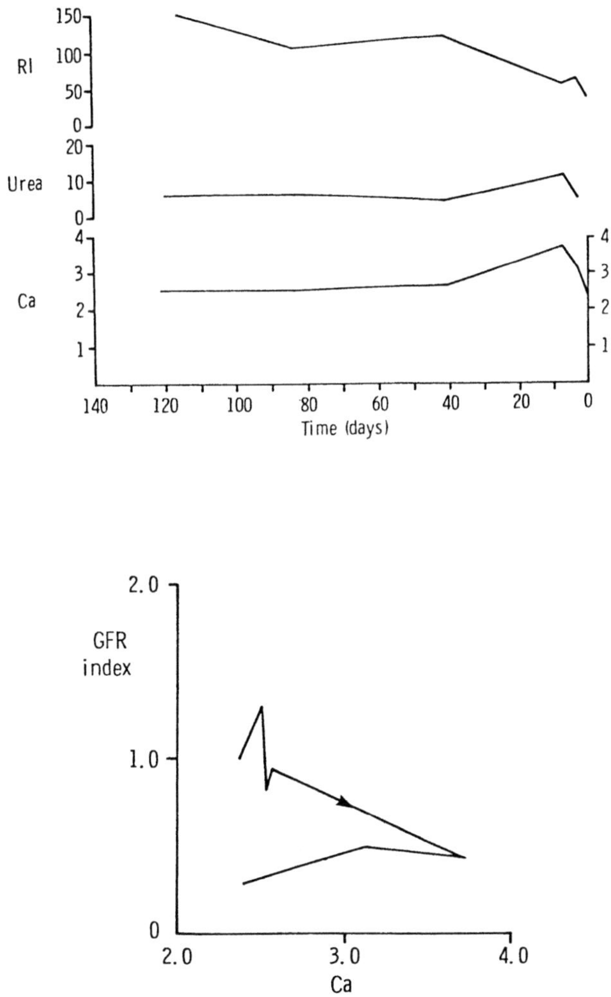

b

(b) This patient's GFR also fell associated with a rise in serum calcium but despite correction of the calcium; renal function continued to deteriorate. RI = renal index (10^4/serum creatinine, μmol/L); urea concentration is in mmol/L; Ca = serum calcium concentration adjusted for albumin (mmol/L); time 0 = day of death; GFR index = serum creatinine concentration as a proportion of that on a day 6 months before death enumerated several effects related to tubular basement membrane morphology followed by cellular destruction and reduced concentrating ability. There was also a low incidence of glycosuria, and, in some patients with hyperparathyroidism, amino aciduria and tubular proteinuria may also occur as discussed subsequently. Glomerular filtration rate also falls with prolonged hypercalcaemia and the effects of antidiuretic hormone are reduced. Recent evidence points to the last factor being due to a direct effect of calcium ions on cyclic adenosine monophosphate production[122,123].

The rate of change in serum calcium is important in that a chronically elevated calcium level is less serious than an acute elevation to the same level and an acute worsening of chronic hypercalcaemia is less severe in its effects than a quantitively similar rise from the normal range[124].

There is histological evidence from animal experiments that an acute rise of calcium levels produces an effect on the proximal tubules with necrosis and sloughing of cells[125,126], although, in the murine model, the levels of calcium associated with this were high, in the order of 4 mmol/L and more[126].

Tubular proteinuria assessed as β_2 microglobulinuria was sought by Wibbell, Dahlberg and Karlsson[127] in ten patients with hyperparathyroidism. Whilst they found three of these patients had β_2 microglobulinuria, it was not related to the serum calcium level, and did not necessarily resolve after parathyroidectomy. These findings are consistent with those of Revillard *et al.*[128] who found no selective tubular proteinuria, although the patterns of pyelonephritis observed may be causally related to nephrocalcinosis. Wibbell *et al.*[127] did, however, identify evidence of distal tubular dysfunction in these patients, manifest by reduced concentrating ability. They concluded that, when hyperparathyroid patients had tubular proteinuria, a cause other than the hypercalcaemia itself should be sought.

In summary, severe hypercalcaemia of acute onset is associated with a reduction of glomular filtration rate which is associated with changes in proximal tubular structure. Chronic hypercalcaemia, however, has less marked effects on renal function and parathyroid hormone may have a protective effect. The kidneys of patients with multiple myeloma seem to be extremely sensitive to hypercalcaemia.

AETIOLOGY OF HYPERCALCAEMIA IN MULTIPLE MYELOMA

Hypercalcaemia is a common complication of malignant disease. The mechanisms known or believed to be responsible for this phenomenon have been enumerated by Besarab and Caro[129]. In some patients, this appears to be mediated by non-humoral processes; in the majority, it is a humoral effect as suggested by the high rate of excretion of nephrogenous cyclic adenosine monophosphate, which resembles that seen in primary hyperparathyroidism[130,131]. Rude *et al.*[132] confirmed that hypercalcaemia of humoral origin is the commoner type.

Haematopoietic tissue has a physiological ability to affect bone[133] and so it is not surprising that haematological disorders may produce an excessive destruction of bone[134] with hypercalcaemia occurring in other conditions besides multiple myeloma[135]. Mundy and colleagues[136,137] have produced evidence that the tumour cells of multiple myeloma produce this osteoclast activating factor (OAF). In contrast to parathyroid hormone, this factor appears to increase osteolytic activity by a mechanism which does not involve adenyl cyclase[138]. The occurrence of bone lesions is associated with increased hydroxyproline excretion which is an indicator of bone catabolism[139]. This is consistent with the observation that the rate of production of OAF reflects disease activity and is related to the extent of osteolytic lesions[23] but there is no direct relationship with serum calcium concentrations. The failure of indices of bone reabsorption to correlate with serum calcium indicates that another factor, such as renal function and calcium excretion, is concerned in the development of hypercalcaemia[115].

Understanding of the development of hypercalcaemia in myeloma patients, therefore, depends to a considerable degree on the understanding of OAF. This is probably not a single entity; increased bone absorption is among the physiological effects of transforming growth factors α and β and of lymphokines, including interleukin 1, lymphotoxin and tumour necrosis factor[140].

SUMMARY

Multiple myeloma is a malignant tumour of plasma cells which is not infrequently seen in clinical practice. Clinical manifestations vary considerably but patients with symptomatic disease benefit from chemotherapy accompanied by supportive measures. The prognosis remains poor and can be assessed by estimates of tumour mass and by the serum β_2 microglobulin. Renal function is impaired in many patients with myeloma and is associated with a poor prognosis. The mechanism of renal impairment depends largely on the toxic effects of free immunoglobulin light chains on the kidney. Hypercalcaemia is a complication of multiple myeloma which arises principally because of increased bone resorption. It compounds the pre-existing light chain effect in causing the deterioration of kidney function.

Acknowledgements

I am grateful to Mrs Ann Thody for her work in preparing the manuscript. Data on patients in West Yorkshire refer to a group observed by me whilst they were under the care of Dr J. A. Child and Professor R. L. Turner, to whom thanks are due.

REFERENCES

1. Clamp, J. R. (1967). Some aspects of the first recorded case of multiple myeloma. *Lancet*, **2,** 1354–1356
2. Bence Jones, H. (1848). On a new substance occurring in the urine of a patient with mollities ossium. *Phil. Trans. R. Soc.*, 55–62
3. Bence Jones, H. (1847). Papers on chemical pathology. Lecture III. *Lancet*, **2,** 88–92
4. Dalrymple, J. (1846). On the microscopical character of mollities ossium. *Dublin J. Med. Sci.*, **2,** 85–95
5. MacIntyre, W. (1850). Case of mollities et fragilitas ossium. *Med. Chir. Trans.*, **33,** 211–232
6. Bayrd, E. D. and Heck, F. J. (1947). Multiple myeloma. A review of 83 proved cases. *J. Am. Med. Assoc.*, **133,** 147–157
7. Salmon, S. E. and Seligmann, M. (1974). B-cell neoplasia in man. *Lancet*, **2,** 1230–1233
8. Pierson, J., Darley, T., Stevenson, G. T. and Virji, M. (1980). Monoclonal immunoglobulin light chains in urine of patients with lymphomas. *Br. J. Cancer*, **41,** 681–688

9. Hobbs, J. R. (1967). Paraproteins – benign or malignant? *Br. Med. J.*, **3,** 699–704
10. Paladini, G., Sala, P. G. and Sautini, P. A. (1980). Benign Bence Jones gammopathy. *Acta Haematol.*, **63,** 241–246
11. Tubbs, R. R., Gephardt, G. N. and McMahon, J. T. (1981). Light chain nephropathy. *Am. J. Med.*, **71,** 263–269
12. Kyle, R. A. (1978). Monoclonal gammopathy of undetermined significance. *Am. J. Med.*, **64,** 814–826
13. Kyle, R. A. and Greipp, P. R. (1982). Idiopathic Bence Jones proteinuria. *N. Engl. J. Med.*, **306,** 564–607
14. Durie, B. G. M. and Salmon, S. E. (1977). Multiple myeloma, macroglobulinaemia and monoclonal gammopathies. In Hoffbrand, A. V., Brainm, M. L. and Hirsch, J. (eds.) *Recent Advances in Haematology 2.* (London: Churchill Livingstone)
15. Chronic Leukaemia–Myeloma Task Force (1973). National Cancer Institute. Proposed guidelines for protocol studies II: Plasma cell myeloma. *Cancer Chemother. Rep.*, **4,** 145–158
16. Parker, D. and Malpas, J. S. (1979). Multiple myeloma. *J. R. Coll. Phys. London,* **13,** 146–153
17. Kyle, R. A. (1975). Multiple myeloma; a review of 869 cases. *Mayo Clin. Proc.*, **50,** 29–40
18. Barteloni, C., Flamini, G. and Logoscino, C. (1980). IgD kappa 'non-secretory' multiple myeloma. Report of a case. *Blood,* **56,** 898–901
19. Kapadia, S. B. (1980). Multiple myeloma: a clinicopathologic study of 62 consecutively autopsied cases. *Medicine* (*Baltimore*), **59,** 380–392
20. Stone, M. J. and Frenkel, E. P. (1975). The clinical spectrum of light chain myeloma. *Am. J. Med.*, **58,** 601–617
21. Pruzanski, W. (1976). Clinical manifestation of multiple myeloma in relation to class and type of M component. *Can. Med. Assoc. J.*, **114,** 898–897
22. Perry, M. and Kyle, R. A. (1975). The clinical significance of Bence Jones proteinuria. *Mayo Clin. Proc.*, **56,** 234–238
23. Durie, B. G. M., Cole, P. W., Chen, H. S. G. *et al.* (1981). Synthesis and metabolism of Bence Jones protein and calculation of tumour burden in patients with Bence Jones myeloma. *Br. J. Haematol.*, **47,** 7–19
24. Gallango, M. C., Swinger, R. and Ramirez, M. (1980). Bence Jones myeloma with a tetramer of kappa type globulin in serum. *Clin. Chem.*, **26,** 1741–1744
25. Roberts-Thompson, P. J., Venables, G. S., Onitiri, A. C. and Leavis, B. (1975). Polymeric IgA myeloma. *Postgrad. Med. J.*, **51,** 44–51
26. Roberts-Thompson, P. J., Mason, D. Y. and MacLennan, I. C. M. (1976). *Br. J. Haematol.*, **33,** 117–130
27. Shustik, C., Bergsagel, D. E. and Pruzanski, W. (1976). Kappa and lambda light chain disease: survival rates and clinical manifestations. *Blood,* **48,** 41–51
28. Velez, R., Beral, V. and Cuzick, J. (1982). Increasing trends of multiple myeloma mortality in England and Wales; 1950–79 are the changes real? *J. Natl. Cancer Inst.*, **69,** 387–392
29. Linos, A., Kyle, R. A. and O'Fahon, L. T. (1981). Incidence and secular trend of multiple myeloma in Olmsted County, Minnesota 1965–1977. *J. Natl. Cancer Inst.*, **66,** 17–20
30. Blattner, W. A. (1980). Epidemiology of multiple myeloma and related plasma

cell disorders. In Potter, M. (ed.) *Progress in Myeloma*, pp. 1–65. (New York: Elsevier)
31. Egan, E. L., Grimes, H. and O'Biern, D. P. (1978). Multiple myeloma in the West of Ireland, presentation and frequency. *Ir. Med. J.*, **71,** 23–26
32. Blattner, W. A., Blair, A. and Mason, T. J. (1981). Multiple myeloma in the United States 1950–1975. *Cancer*, **48,** 2547–2554
33. Durie, B. G. M. and Salmon, S. E. (1975). A clinical staging system for multiple myeloma. *Cancer*, **36,** 842–854
34. Woodruff, R. K., Wadsworth, J., Malpas, J. S. and Tobias, J. S. (1979). Clinical staging in multiple myeloma. *Br. J. Haematol.*, **42,** 199–205
35. Salmon, S. E. and Wampler, S. B. (1978). Multiple myeloma. Quantitative staging and assessment of response with a programmable pocket calculator. *Blood*, **49,** 379–389
36. Durie, B. G. M., Cole, P. W., Chen, H. S. G. *et al.* (1981). Synthesis and metabolism of Bence Jones protein and calculation of tumour burden in patients with Bence Jones myeloma. *Br. J. Haematol.*, **47,** 7–19
37. Medical Research Council (1973). Report on the first myelomatosis trial Part I. Analysis of presenting features of prognostic importance. *Br. J. Haematol.*, **24,** 123–139
38. Medical Research Council (1980). Prognostic features in the third MRC myelomatosis trial. *Br. J. Cancer*, **42,** 831
39. Peto, R. (1971). Myeloma workshop: Urea, albumin and response rates. *Br. Med. J.*, **1,** 324
40. Alexanian, R., Balcerzak, S., Bonner, J. D. *et al.* (1975). Prognostic features of multiple myeloma. *Cancer*, **36,** 1192–1201
41. Matzner, Y., Benbassat, J. and Polliack, A. (1978). Prognostic factors in multiple myeloma. *Acta Haematol.*, **60,** 257–268
42. Colls, B. M. and Barlow, B. A. (1979). Multiple myeloma – prognosis, treatment and survival in an 8 year study. *Aust. N.Z. J. Med.*, **9,** 262–268
43. Durie, B. G. M., Salmon, S. E. and Moon, T. E. (1980). Pretreatment tumour mass in multiple myeloma. *Blood*, **55,** 364–372
44. Jansen, J., Huijgens, P. L. and Van der Velde, E. A. (1980). Prognosis of multiple myeloma. *Neth. Med. J.*, **13,** 246–251
45. Merlini, G., Waldenstrom, J. C. and Jagakar, S. D. (1980). A new improved clinical staging system for multiple myeloma based on analysis of 123 treated patients. *Blood*, **55,** 1011–1019
46. Johannsson, B. (1971). Prognostic features in mvelomatosis. *Br. Med. J.*, **1,** 327–
47. Cornell, C. J., McIntyre, O. R., Kochwa, S. *et al.* (1979). Response to therapy in IgG myeloma patients excreting or light chains. CALGB experience. *Blood*, **54,** 23–29
48. Graham, R. C. and Bernier, G. M. (1975). The bone marrow in multiple myeloma. *Medicine* (*Baltimore*), **54,** 225–243
49. Latreille, J., Barlogie, B., Johnson, D. *et al.* (1982). Ploidy and proliferative characteristics in monoclonal gammopathies. *Blood*, **59,** 43–51
50. Gassmann, W., Pralle, H., Haferlach, T. *et al.* (1985). Staging systems for multiple myeloma: a comparison. *Br. J. Haematol.*, **59,** 703–711
51. Norfolk, D. R., Child, J. A., Cooper, E. H. *et al.* (1980). Serum beta$_2$ microglobulin in myelomatosis. Potential value in stratification and monitoring. *Br. J. Cancer*, **42,** 510–515

52. Morrell, A. and Riesen, W. (1980). Serum beta$_2$ microglobulin serum creatinine and bone marrow plasma cell count in benign and malignant monoclonal gammopathy. *Acta Haematol.*, **64,** 87–93
53. Bataille, R., Magub, M., Sany, J. *et al.* (1981). Beta^2 microglobuline serique au cours du myelome multiple. *Rev. Rheum.*, **48,** 235–240
54. Bataille, R., Magub, M., Grenier, J., Donnadio, D. and Sany, J. (1981). Serum beta$_2$ microglobulin in multiple myeloma. Relation to presenting features and clinical status. *Eur. J. Cancer Clin.*, **18,** 59–66
55. Child, J. A., Crawford, S. M., Norfolk, D. R. *et al.* (1983). Evaluation of serum beta$_2$ microglobulin as a prognostic indicator in myelomatosis. *Br. J. Cancer*, **47,** 111–114
56. Cuzick, J., Cooper, E. H. and MacLennan, I. C. M. (1985). The prognostic value of serum beta$_2$ microglobulin compared with other presentation features in myelomatosis. *Br. J. Cancer*, **52,** 1–6
57. van Dobbenburgh, O. A., Rodenhuis, S., Ockhuizen, T. *et al.* (1985). Serum beta$_2$ microglobulin: a real improvement in the management of multiple myeloma? *Br. J. Haematol*, **61,** 611–620.
58. Colls, B. M. and Darlow, B. A. (1979). Multiple myeloma – prognosis, treatment and survival in an 8 year study. *Aust. N.Z. J. Med.*, **9,** 262–268
59. Alexanian, R., Fraschini, G. and Smith, L. (1984). Amyloidosis in multiple myeloma or without apparent cause. *Arch. Int. Med.*, **144,** 2158–2160
60. Buckman, R., Cuzick, J. and Galton, D. A. G. (1982). Long-term survival in myelomatosis. *Br. J. Haematol.*, **52,** 589–599
61. Alexanian, R. (1985). Ten year survival in multiple myeloma. *Arch. Int. Med.*, **145,** 2073–2074
62. Jeffries, D. J. (1985). Clinical use of acyclovir. *Br. Med. J.*, **290,** 177–178
63. Harris, D. C. H., Ibels, L. S., Ravich, R. B. M., Isbister, J. P. and Wells, J. V. (1983). Multiple myeloma with renal failure, a case for intensive treatment. *Aust. N.Z. J. Med.*, **13,** 163–167
64. Coward, R. A., Mallick, N. P. and Delamore, I. W. (1983). Should patients with renal failure associated with myeloma be dialized? *Br. Med. J.*, **287,** 1575–1578
65. Medical Research Council working party on leukaemia in adults (1984). Analysis and management of renal failure in fourth MRC myelomatosis trial. *Br. Med. J.*, **288,** 1411–1416
66. Clyne, D. H., Pesce, A. J. and Thompson, R. E. (1979). Nephrotoxicity of Bence Jones Protein in the rat: Importance of protein isoelectric point. *Kidney Int.*, **16,** 345–352
67. Johns, E. A., Turner, R., Cooper, E. H. and MacLennan, I. C. M. (1986). Isoelectric points of urinary light chains in myelomatosis; analysis in relation to nephrotoxicity. *J. Clin Pathol.*, **39,** 833–837
68. Medical Research Council working party on leukaemia in adults (1985). Objective evaluation of the role of vincristine in induction and maintenance therapy for myelomatosis. *Br. J. Cancer*, **52,** 153–158
69. Bergsagel, D. E. (1985). Controversies in the treatment of plasma cell myeloma. *Postgrad. Med. J.*, **61,** 109–116
70. Hyrniuk, W. and Bush, H. (1986). The importance of dose intensity in chemotherapy of metastatic breast cancer. *J. Clin. Oncol.*, **2,** 1281–1288
71. MacLennan I. C. M. (1987). Personal communication.
72. Barlogie, B., Hall, R., Zander, A., Dicke, K. and Alexanian, R. (1986). High

dose melphalan with autologous bone marrow transplantation for multiple myeloma. *Blood*, **67**, 1298–1301
73. Selby, P., McElwain, T. J., Nandi, A. A. *et al.* (1987). Multiple myeloma treated with high dose intravenous melphalan. *Br. J. Haematol.*, **66**, 55–62
74. Barlogie, B., Smith, L. and Alexanian, R. (1984). Effective treatment of advanced multiple myeloma refractory to alkylating agents. *N. Engl. J. Med.*, **310**, 1353–1356
75. Alexanian, R., Barlogie, B. and Dixon, D. (1986). High dose glucocorticoid treatment of resistant myeloma. *Ann. Int. Med.*, **195**, 8–11
76. Ohno, R. and Kimara, K. (1986). Treatment of multiple myeloma with recombinant interferon alpha 2a. *Cancer*, **57**, 1685–1688
77. Case, D. C., Sonneborn, H. C., Paul, S. D. *et al.* (1986). Phase II study of r-DNA alpha 2 interferon (intron A) in patients with multiple myeloma utilising an escalating induction phase. *Cancer Treat. Rep.*, **70**, 1251–1254
78. Thomas, P. J., Daban, A. and Bontoux, D. (1984). Double hemibody irradiation in chemotherapy resistant multiple myeloma. *Cancer Treat. Rep.*, **68**, 1173–1175
79. Tobias, J. S., Richards, J. D., Blackman, G. M., Joannides, T., Trask, C. W. and Nathan, J. I. (1985). Hemibody irradiation in multiple myeloma. *Radiother. Oncol.*, **3**, 11–16
80. Hobbs, J. R. (1975). Monitoring myelomatosis. *Arch. Int. Med.*, **135**, 125–130
81. Hobbs, J. R. (1971). Mode of escape from therapeutic control in myelomatosis. *Br. Med. J.*, **1**, 325
82. Cohen, H. J., Bartolucci, A. A., Forman, W. B. and Silberman, H. R. (1986). Consolidation and maintenance therapy in multiple myeloma: randomised comparison of a new approach to therapy after initial response to treatment. *J. Clin. Oncol.*, **4**, 888–899
83. Crawford, S. M. (1985). Hypercalcaemia, renal failure and relapse in multiple myeloma. *Cancer*, **55**, 898–900
84. Bell, E. T. (1933). Renal lesions associated with multiple myeloma. *Am. J. Pathol.*, **9**, 393–419
85. Foord, A. G. and Randall, L. (1935). Hyperproteinaemia, Autohaemaglutination and renal insufficiency in multiple myeloma. *Am. J. Clin. Pathol.*, **5**, 532–547
86. Blackman, S. S., Halsey Barker, W., Buell. M. V. and Davis, B. D. (1944). On the pathogenesis of renal failure associated with multiple myeloma. *J. Clin. Invest.*, **23**, 163–166
87. Rota, S., Mougenot, B., Bandoin, B. *et al.* (1987). Multiple myeloma and severe renal failure; a clinicopathologic study of outcome and prognosis in 34 patients. *Medicine*, **66**, 126–137
88. Cohen, A. H. and Border, W. A. (1980). Myeloma kidney: An immunomorphogenetic study of renal biopsies. *Lab. Invest.*, **42**, 248–256
89. Border, W. A. and Cohen, A. H. (1980). Renal biopsy of clinically silent multiple myeloma. *Ann. Int. Med.*, **93**, 43–46
90. Abrahams, C., Pirani, C. C. and Pollak, V. E. (1966). Ultrastructure of the kidney in a patient with multiple myeloma. *J. Pathol. Bact.*, **92**, 220–224
91. Sirota, J. H. and Hamerman, D. (1954). Renal function studies in an adult subject with the Fanconi syndrome. *Am. J. Med.*, **16**, 138–145
92. Maldonado, J. E., Velosa, J. A. and Kyle, R. A. *et al.* (1975). Fanconi syndrome in adults. *Am J. Med.*, **58**, 354–363

93. Walb, D., Wohlenberg, H., Rampelt, H.J., Schmider, H. and Thomas, L. (1980). Fanconi syndrom des Erwachsenen bei Fruhymelom mit monokloner gammopathie IgG. Typ. Kappa. *Deutsche Med. Wochenschrift*, **195,** 1355–1359
94. Finkel, P. N., Kronentarg, K., Pesce, A. J. *et al.* (1973). Adult Fanconi syndrome, amyloidosis and marked kappa chain proteinuria. *Nephron*, **10,** 1–24
95. Rawlings, W., Griffin, J., Duffy, T. and Humphrey, R. (1975). Fanconi syndrome with lambda light chains in urine. *N. Engl. J. Med.*, **292,** 1315
96. De Fronzo, R.A., Cooke, C.R., Wright, J.R. and Humphrey, R.C. (1978). Renal function in patients with multiple myeloma. *Medicine* (*Baltimore*), **57,** 151–166
97. Smithline, N., Kassirer, J. P. and Cohen, J. J. (1976). Light chain nephropathy – renal tubular dysfunction associated with light chain proteinuria. *N. Engl. J. Med.*, **294,** 71–74
98. Sanchez, L. M. and Domz, C. A. (1960). Renal patterns in myeloma. *Ann. Int. Med.*, **52,** 44–54
99. Lazar, G. S. and Feinstein, D. I. (1981). Distal renal tubular acidosis in multiple myeloma. *Arch. Int. Med.*, **141,** 655–657
100. Forbus, W. D., Perlzweig, W. A. and Parfentier, I. A. (1935). Bence Jones protein excretion and its effects upon the kidney. *Bull. Johns Hopkins Hosp.*, **57,** 47–69
101. Rees, E. G. and Waugh, W. H. (1965). Factors in the renal failure of multiple myeloma. *Arch. Int. Med.*, **116,** 400–405
102. Martinez-Maldonado, M., Yiam, T., Suki, W. N. and Erehogan, G. (1971). Renal complications in multiple myeloma: Pathophysiology and some aspects of clinical management. *J. Chron. Dis.*, **24,** 221–237
103. Schubert, G. E., Veigel, J. and Lennert, K. (1972). Structure and function of kidney in multiple myeloma. *Virchow's Arch. Pathol. Anat.*, **355,** 135–157
104. Clyne, D. H., Brendstrup, L., First, M. R. *et al.* (1974). Renal effects of intraperitoneal kappa chain injection. *Lab. Invest.*, **2,** 131–142
105. Beaufils, M. and Morel-Maroger, L. (1978). Pathogenesis of renal disease in monoclonal gammopathies. Current concepts. *Nephron*, **30,** 125–131
106. Cooper, E. H., Forbes, M. A., Crockson, R. A. and MacLennan, I. C. M. (1984). Proximal renal tubular function in myelomatosis: observations in the fourth Medical Research Council trial. *J. Clin. Pathol.*, **37,** 852–858
107. Randall, R. E., Williamson, W. C., Mallinson, F., Tuny, M. Y. and Still, W. J. S. (1976). Manifestations of systemic light chain deposition. *Am. J. Med.*, **60,** 293–299
108. Scully, R. E., Galdabini, J. and McNeely, B. U. (1981). Case records of Massachusetts General Hospital. *N. Engl. J. Med.*, **304,** 33–43
109. Seymour, S. E., Thompson, A. J., Smith, P. S., Woodroffe, A. J. and Clarkson, A. R. (1980). Kappa light chain clomerulosclerosis in multiple myeloma. *Am. J. Pathol.*, **101,** 557–580
110. Solling, K., Solling, J. and Jacobsen, O. (1980). Non-secretory myeloma associated with nodular glomerulosclerosis. *Acta Med. Scand.*, **207,** 137–143
111. Van Geelan, J. A. and Mulder, A. W. (1979). Histology and function of the kidney in marked Bence Jones proteinuria. *Neth. J. Med.*, **22,** 158–160
112. Nagengast, F. M., Assmann, K. J. M. and Fennis, J. F. M. (1980). Histology and function of the kidney in marked Bence Jones proteinuria. *Neth. J. Med.*, **23,** 38

113. Koss, M. N., Pirani, C. L. and Osserman, E. F. (1976). Experimental Bence Jones cast nephropathy. *Lab. Invest.*, **34,** 579–591
114. De Fronzo, R. A., Humphrey, R. C., Wright, J. R. and Cooke, C. R. (1975). Acute renal failure in multiple myeloma. *Medicine* (*Baltimore*), **54,** 209–223
115. Heyburn, P. J., Child, J. A. and Peacock, M. (1981). Relative importance of renal failure and increased bone resorption in the hypercalcaemia of myelomatosis. *J. Clin. Pathol.*, **34,** 54–57
16. Vavatsi-Manos, O. and Preuss, H. G. (1976). The effects of high calcium concentrations on renal ammoniagenesis by the kidney slices. *Nephron*, **17,** 474–484
17. Vanherweghem, J. L., Docobu, J., D'Jollander, A. and Toussaint, C. (1976). Effect of hypercalcaemia on water and sodium excretion by the isolated kidney. *Pflug. Arch.*, **363,** 75–80
118. Nutbeam, H. M., Sinclair, L. and Oberholger, V. G. (1979). Magnesium transport deficit with hypercalcaemia. *J. R. Soc. Med.*, **72,** 932–934
119. Parfitt, A. M. and Kleerekoper, M. (1980). Clinical disorders of calcium phosphorus and magnesium metabolism. In Maxwell, M. H. and Kleeman, C. R. (eds.) *Clinical Disorders of Fluid and Electrolyte Metabolism*, 3rd Edn. (New York: McGraw Hill)
120. Humes, H. D. (1986). Role of calcium in pathogenesis of acute renal failure. *Am. J. Physiol.*, **250,** F579–F589
121. Epstein, F. H. (1968). Calcium and the kidney. *Am. J. Med.*, **45,** 700–714
122. Takaichi, K., Uchida, S. and Kurokawa, K. (1986). High Ca^{2+} inhibit a AVP dependent cAMP production in thick ascending limbs of Henle. *Am. J. Physiol.*, **250,** F770–7706
123. Teitelbaum, I. and Berl, T. (1986). Effects of calcium on vasopressin mediated cyclic adenosine monophosphate formation in cultured rat inner medullary tubule cells. *J. Clin Invest.*, **77,** 1574–1583
124. Benabe, J. E. and Martinez-Maldonado, M. (1978). Hypercalaemic nephropathy. *Arch. Int. Med.*, **138,** 777–779
125. Duffy, J. L., Suzuki, Y. and Churg, J. (1971). Acute calcium nephropathy. *Arch. Pathol.*, **91,** 340–350
126. Ganote, C. E., Philipsborn, D. S., Chen, E. and Carone, F. A. (1975). Acute calcium nephrotoxicity. *Arch. Pathol.*, **99,** 650–657
127. Wibbell, L., Dahlberg, P. A. and Karlsson, A. (1974). Hyperparathyroidism associated with distal tubular dysfunction. *Acta Med. Scand.*, **206,** 507–510
128. Revillard, J. P., Manuel, Y., Francois, R. and Traeger, J. (1970). Renal disease associated with tubular proteinuria. In Manuel, Y., Revillard, J. P. and Betael, H. (eds.) *Protein in Normal and Pathological Urine*. (Basel: Karger)
129. Besarab, A. and Caro, J. (1978). Mechanism of hypercalcaemia in malignancy. *Cancer*, **41,** 2276–2285
130. Stewart, A. F., Horst, R., Deftos, L. J. *et al.* (1980). Biochemical evaluation of patients with cancer associated hypercalcaemia. *N. Engl. J. Med.*, **303,** 1377–1383
131. Werner, S. and Low, H. (1977). Urinary excretion of CAMP and GMP in primary hyperparathyroidism with reference to clinical signs and symptoms. *Horm. Metab. Res.*, **9,** 332–336
132. Rude, R. K., Sharp, C. F., Fredericko, R. S. *et al.* (1981). Urinary and nephrogenous adenosine 3′5′ monophosphate in the hypercalcaemia of malignancy. *J. Clin. Endothel. Metab.*, **52,** 765–771

133. Raisz, L. G. (1981). What marrow does to bone. *N. Engl. J. Med.*, **304,** 1485–1486
134. Pootrakul, P., Hungsprenges, S. and Fucharoen, S. (1981). Relation between erythropoiesis and bone metabolism in thalassaemia. *N. Engl. J. Med.*, **304,** 1470–1473
135. Walter, R. M. and Greenberg, B. R. (1980). Hypercalcaemia in the accelerated phase of chronic myelogenous leukaemia. *Cancer*, **46,** 1174–1178
136. Mundy, G. R., Luber, R. A., Raisz, L. G. *et al.* (1974). Bone resorbing activity in supernatant from lymphoid cell lines. *N. Engl. J. Med.*, **290,** 867–871
137. Mundy, G. R., Raisz, L. G. and Cooper, R. A. *et al.* (1974). Evidence for the secretion of an osteoclast stimulating factor in myeloma. *N. Engl. J. Med.*, **291,** 1041–1046
138. Josse, R. G., Murray, T. M., Mundy, G. R. *et al.* (1981). Observations on the mechanisms of bone resorption induced by multiple myeloma culture fluids and partially purified osteoclast activating factor. *J. Clin. Invest.*, **67,** 1472–1481
139. Niel, H. B., Neely, C. L. and Palmieri, G. M. (1981). The postabsorption urinary hydrolyproline (Spot HYPRO) in patients with multiple myeloma. *Cancer*, **48,** 783–787
140. Mundy, G. R. (1987). The hypercalcaemia of malignancy. *Kidney Int.*, **31,** 142–155

3

LUPUS NEPHRITIS

F. W. BALLARDIE

INTRODUCTION

Nephritis in systemic lupus erythematosus represents the archetype of variable organ involvement of a disease. Our knowledge of the natural history of lupus nephritis has significantly improved in the last decade. There has been continuing refinement in histological classification, coupled with the recognition that the morphologically distinct glomerulopathies can have features of prognostic significance in common. Studies have demonstrated efficacy of immunosuppressive drugs in preserving renal function and reducing renal scarring, but consensus is lacking on the precise way in which the therapeutic regimes should be used. Most analyses have used either end-stage renal failure or death as a measure of outcome. Yet, the most common problems with which the clinician is faced are optimizing treatment of chronic, indolent or inactive disease whilst attempting to prevent the acute, possibly life-threatening flares of systemic lupus with nephritis. Recognition that acute deterioration in renal function in lupus nephritis is common proves the necessity for vigilance in management of each phase of the disease and indicates the need for a detailed, sensitive interpretation of the therapeutic needs of the individual patient.

This chapter will focus on aspects of the literature which contribute most to our understanding of clinical disease resulting from the lupus glomerulopathies. Consideration will be made of evolving concepts of the immunopathogenesis of the nephritides. Widely regarded as the prototype immune complex disease, recent findings have challenged this concept. Circulating anti-DNA antibodies have been shown to be cross reactive with intrinsic glomerular antigens and connective tissue components distributed throughout basement membranes in the body. This suggests the possibility that the morphologically distinct lupus glomerulopathies are the result of an autoimmune process, from deposition of antibodies directed against intrinsic renal antigens. The need is evident for continuing reappraisal of our perception of the pathogenesis of the lupus glomerulopathies. Further developments in the management of lupus nephritis are likely to follow such a re-evaluation. Major outstanding problems – the role of plasma exchange, the reasons for continued mortality – will also be stressed so that the physician may further rationalize and optimize his clinical approach to lupus nephritis.

RENAL INVOLVEMENT IN SYSTEMIC LUPUS ERYTHEMATOSUS

Diagnosis

Establishing the diagnosis of SLE in most cases is uncomplicated. The preliminary criteria of the American Rheumatism Association, revised in 1982[1], include as alternatives to the LE cell phenomenon antibodies to native DNA or the extractable nuclear antigen, Sm (Table 3.1). Although 90% of patients with systemic lupus have positive antinuclear antibodies, the diagnosis does not depend on laboratory tests. The critera have high specificity and sensitivity in establishing a diagnosis of SLE, distinct from other collagen vascular diseases.

Detection and development of nephritis

Nephritis is common in SLE, perhaps invariable. Its definition is dependent on policy for renal biopsy. Clinical evidence of nephritis, defined by significant proteinuria, abnormal urinary sediment or renal dysfunction, is present in 10% of adult patients with SLE at presentation, but will develop in about two of every three patients during the course of their disease[2]. Renal biopsy performed on patients without clinical evidence of nephritis reveals a significant further number of renal lesions – even severe diffuse proliferative glo-

TABLE 3.1 The revised criteria for classification of SLE

(1)	Malar	Rash
(2)	Discoid	Rash
(3)	Photosensitivity	Rash
(4)	Oral ulcers	
(5)	Arthritis	
(6)	Serositis	
(7)	Nephritis:	proteinuria > 0.5 g/day abnormal urinary sediment
(8)	Central nervous system disorder:	seizures psychosis
(9)	Haematological disorder:	haemolysis leucopaenia thrombocytopaenia
(10)	Immunological disorder:	LE cell anti-DNA/Sm
(11)	Antinuclear antibody	

The presence of 4 or more criteria constitutes SLE (Ref. 1). Immunological criteria (10) and/or (11) are generally considered a prerequisite for the diagnosis

merulonephritis – the 'silent nephritis' of SLE[3,4]. The effects of subclinical nephritis on longer term renal function and glomerular scarring are not known, but this important finding warrants further analysis. Therapy at this stage could influence the subsequent development of overt nephritis or progressive scarring. Radioimmunoassay of urine, normal in conventional assay, can show microalbuminuria in lupus patients[5]. Steroid therapy suppresses this abnormality. The physician responsible for a patient with systemic lupus in the general medical or rheumatological clinic should therefore perform a urinalysis on each attendance to detect clinical disease at an early stage.

The variable association of nephritis in some patients with disease of other systems in SLE[6] is perplexing, and may prove to be fundamental in the pathogenesis of organ injury.

Clinical associations

The modes of presentation of lupus with clinically evident nephritis are typical of SLE as a whole[7]. Commonly, more than one feature is present. Arthritis is most frequently the major symptom[8] with rash, pleurisy and thrombocytopaenia in the minority. Proteinuria in the nephrotic range is present in more than half the cases, but rapidly progressive renal failure is infrequent. Although SLE is very much less common in males, the clinical expression of disease has many similarities to that in females[9]. Renal involvement is similar, but central nervous system disease dominates in females while pleurisy is common in males.

Episodic acute deteriorations in renal function with extrarenal manifestations are again common – averaging 1.6 features per episode[10]. Central nervous system disorders dominate the clinical picture, however. It is also clear that severe nephritis may be unaccompanied by extrarenal manifestations in individuals, even though the patient has previously suffered symptomatic SLE without clinical evidence of nephritis. Such transitions in the clinical expression of organ involvement in SLE merit constant vigilance.

In contrast to this typical pattern of onset of renal disease, it is clear that glomerulonephritis can herald the later diagnosis of SLE[6]. Clinical evidence of renal disease, with glomerular lesions indistinguishable on morphology, immunohistology, and electron microscopy, from those in unequivocal cases of SLE, may precede by several years the clinical and serological definition of SLE.

Functional implications of renal biopsy findings: Natural history of lupus nephritis

Recognition that wide variations in renal morphology occur in SLE, both between patients and in longitudinal studies of individuals with repeated biopsies, has presented a complex problem of defining influences on outcome in long-term studies (Table 3.2). Whilst attempts have been made to formulate prognostic indices – identifying specific clinical, serological, or histological features which correlate with prognosis[11,12] – some early studies suggested no difference between the morphologically distinct glomerulopathies in the likelihood of developing end–stage renal failure[8]. Although progressive renal failure does not usually accompany lupus nephritis classes I and II, caution is required in follow-up of patients with these renal lesions. Membranous lupus nephropathy, initially considered a benign lesion in SLE[13] has a course similar to that of idiopathic membranous nephropathy, with progressive disease in a minority[14].

TABLE 3.2 Basic WHO classification of lupus glomerulonephropathies[7]

Class	*Glomerulonephritis*	*Microscopy*		
		Light	*Immunofluorescence: Immunoglobulin + complement*	*EM*
I	Minimal change	Normal	0	0
II	Mesangial, proliferative	Mesangial expansion and/or hypercellularity	M > En, C	M > En
III	Focal and segmental, proliferative	Mesangial proliferative with segmental intracapillary proliferation	M > En, C	M > En
IV	Diffuse, proliferative	Diffuse hypercellularity, mesangial interposition, thrombi crescents	M, En, C, Ep (intense staining)	M, En, Ep
V	Membranous	Basement membrane thickening, spikes Variable mesangial hypercellularity	M, Ep > C, En	M,Ep > C
—	Interstial nephritis	Interstitial inflammatory cell infiltrate	Tubular basement membrane	

Subclasses are recognized.
Immunofluorescence and electron microscopy: M = mesangial; C = capillary wall; En = subendothelial; Ep = subepithelial.
Interstitial nephritis is also a recognized association of SLE

It is now generally considered that diffuse proliferative glomerulonephritis (WHO class IV) carries the worst renal prognosis[14,15]. The lesion may herald the later development of necrotizing vasculitis with glomerular crescent formation[2] and rapidly progressive intractable acute renal failure. Mortality is highest in the group of patients with diffuse proliferative glomerulonephritis (Figure 3.1).

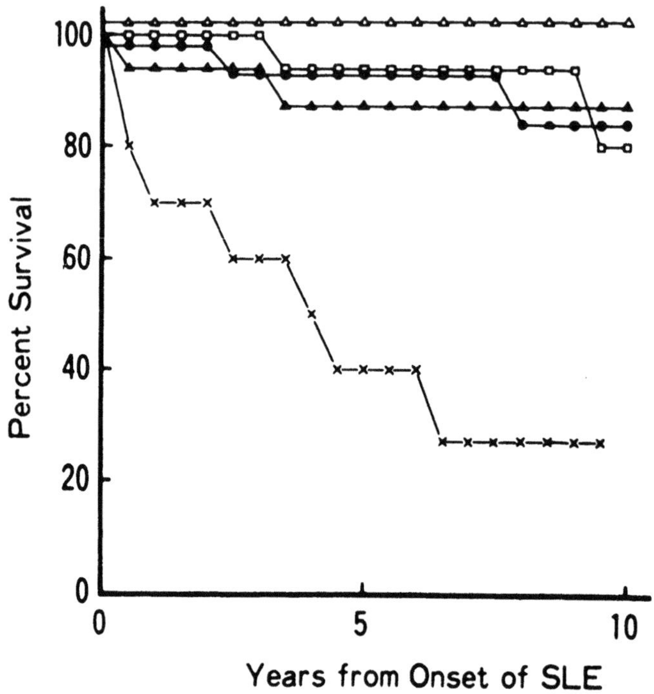

FIGURE 3.1 Cumulative patient survival from onset of SLE-associated glomerulopathies: ● membranous; □ mesangial proliferative; diffuse proliferative – △ mild; ▲ moderate; × severe. (Reproduced from Ref. 15 with permission)

Although the degree of proteinuria, as a measure of renal injury is considered a poor prognostic feature[19], earlier analyses perhaps surprisingly, suggested a tendency towards improved survival in the presence of heavy proteinuria[8]. Nephrotic syndrome most often accompanies diffuse proliferative glomerulonephritis and membranous nephropathy. Proteinuria is milder with mesangial proliferative lesions (Table 3.3) and the implication therefore, is that heavy proteinuria is associated with glomerular lesions which have a worse prognosis.

The presence of scarring and chronic morphological changes, particularly tubular atrophy, also indicates a greater risk of progressive renal failure[16,17] since the pathological processes leading to their formation are least amenable to therapeutic intervention. The extent of

TABLE 3.3 Clinicopathological correlations in lupus nephritis

Clinical	Nephropathy (WHO Class)			
	I and II	III	IV	V
No clinical nephritis	40%	30%	25%	25%
Renal dysfunction:				
Severe: nephrotic/renal failure	<1%	8%	70%	22%
Mild: microscopic haematuria/proteinuria <5 g	10%	21%	63%	6%

Adapted from Ref. 19 with permission

TABLE 3.4 Glomerular morphology evaluated in a semiquantitative scoring system[20]

Activity	Chronicity
Glomerular cell proliferation	Glomerular sclerosis
Leucocyte exudation	Fibrous crescents
Fibrinoid necrosis*	Tubular atrophy
Cellular crescents*	Interstitial fibrosis
Hyaline deposits	
Interstitial mononuclear cell infiltrate	

Features marked * are weighted by a factor of two because of their ominous prognostic significance

proliferative and scarring processes, whatever the initial renal morphology, assessed on a scoring system, provides a semiquantitative method of evaluating the evolution of glomerular morphological changes and their response to treatment (Table 3.4).

A further simplifying interpretation of the significance of renal biopsy findings has been proposed[15], relating the extent of subendothelial deposits on electron microscopy to outcome, independent of the light-microscopic appearances. These deposits were extensive in cases of severe diffuse proliferative nephritis, correlated with activity of SLE and were thus of grave prognostic significance. This view is however, not shared by all investigators[18].

Tubulointerstitial deposits of immunoglobulins and complement, usually with histological evidence of injury, are found in association with glomerular disease. Rarely, the tubulointerstitial changes are the major abnormality on biopsy and linear tubular basement membrane immunoglobulin deposits, or interstitial microcalcification may be present. The tubulointerstitial lupus nephropathies manifest as low-grade proteinuria, possibly accompanied by renal failure or renal tubular acidosis. The renal dysfunction of these nephropathies can be steroid responsive.

The natural history of untreated renal disease in SLE in now difficult to determine. Since studies published over 20 years ago reported 4-year survival of 55% of untreated patients[11], therapeutic intervention, often in uncontrolled studies, has been introduced in most clinico-pathological series. There is general agreement that the prognosis has improved as a consequence[8] and interest is now centred on questions of optimizing therapy for lupus nephritis.

Transformations in lupus nephritis

Change in the renal morphology occurs in 15% of patients with lupus nephritis[2,14]. In most cases, an ostensibly benign lesion transforms to diffuse proliferative glomerulonephritis of variable severity. The episode may be accompanied by renal dysfunction and can be responsible for deterioration in glomerular filtration in individuals with lupus nephropathy.

Acute deteriorations

Progressive renal failure in SLE is not usually considered as a stepwise phenomenon[10]. Episodes of acute renal dysfunction are reported in 18% of lupus nephritis and occur most frequently in the first 12 months after initial presentation, but also at any time subsequently. The differential diagnosis of their cause is that of any potentially

TABLE 3.5 Causes of acute renal dysfunction in lupus nephritis

1.	Rapidly progressive glomerulonephritis
2.	Haemodynamics – volume depletion
3.	Thrombosis – renal vein
	– micro/macro arterial
4.	Infection
5.	Infection + rapidly progressive glomerulonephritis

acute glomerulonephritis (Table 3.5) and each patient requires careful assessment before starting appropriate treatment. Since the precise time course of deterioration is often not known, a general approach is appropriate to define whether the SLE is active, suggesting the presence of glomerulonephritis, or whether a haemodynamic or thrombotic event is the cause. It is often difficult to exclude the possibility of thrombotic events. Doppler ultrasound, dynamic computer tomographic scanning with contrast injection, as well as venography have all been advocated. In the absence of formal comparison of their efficacy in detecting renal vein thrombosis, their use and interpretation depends on local expertise and availability of technique. Arteriography with venous phase imaging of the renal veins is likely to provide fewest false positives and negatives but should be undertaken only after careful consideration.

TREATMENT OF LUPUS NEPHRITIS

The problem of therapy for lupus nephritis has, perhaps, fostered the most capricious regimens and controversy in medicine. The reader is referred to the excellent review of Wagner[21] for a summary of the balance of opinion a decade ago on the merits of immunosuppressive therapy for lupus nephritis. The heterogeneity of disease and numbers of patients in individual centres has contributed to lack of consistency in conclusions between studies. A pooled analysis has been published recently, of all clinical trials in which patients have been randomly assigned to receive either prednisolone or prednisolone plus cyclophosphamide or azathioprine[22]. The conclusion supports the efficacy of immunosuppressive therapy added to prednisolone in preserving renal function in lupus nephritis (Table 3.6), particularly in patients with diffuse proliferative glomerulonephritis.

TABLE 3.6 Summary of the benefits of prednisolone combined with cytotoxic therapy (azathioprine or cyclophosphamide) over steroids alone in lupus nephritis[22]. Significance levels were higher with diffuse proliferative nephritis, suggesting increased benefit from cytotoxic therapy in patients with this glomerular lesion. There was a possible trend with other glomerulopathies

	All studies	*Diffuse proliferative GN*	
	Steroids alone (S) *Combined therapy (C)*	*with* (S) (C)	*without* (S) (C)
Renal deterioration	*	*	N.S.
ESRF	*	*	N.S.
Deaths:			
nephritis related	*	*	N.S.
all	(*)	N.S.	N.S.

* denotes significance, $p<0.05$; (*) $p=0.06$; N.S. – not significant

Such analyses may be of limited value. Improvements in clinical practice with time and between centres cannot be considered. They give evidence for long-term benefit and support the careful use of potentially toxic agents but provide only part of the background necessary in selecting an optimal therapy for an individual patient.

Therapeutic regimens

It is clear that particular categories of patients with lupus nephritis benefit from appropriate use of cytotoxic drugs in terms of preservation of renal function and reduced mortality. Use of these drugs has to be considered in two distinct phases of the treatment of lupus: the management of acute severe life-threatening disease and the long-term management of chronic, indolent or inactive disease. The regimen outlined is that currently used in a number of centres in treating adults with lupus nephritis.

Treatment of the acute phase

Steroids are given initially as oral prednisolone, 60 mg per day for 10 days, with azathioprine, 2.5 mg kg^{-1} day^{-1}. Steroid dose is reduced every 10 days, in 15 mg then 10 mg steps, to 20 mg per day, provided there is improvement in the patients condition. Where there is severe diffuse proliferative nephritis, with crescents, vasculitis, and/or cerebral lupus, cyclophosphamide, 2–2.5 mg/kg is substituted for azathioprine. In these cases, cyclophosphamide is changed back to azathioprine when evidence of lupus activity has diminished. Eight weeks therapy with cyclophosphamide at the doses outlined will, in general, keep the total dose below 8 g and thus minimise the risk of gonadal toxicity.

These are broad guidelines only. The important balance for the physician to achieve is to minimise immunosuppression and exposure to cytotoxic and steroid therapy while at the same time suppressing disease activity. Many tend to underestimate the need for immunosuppressive therapy. Variations in the approach of individual physicians are the major reason why large multicentre analyses do not provide detailed rewarding information on patient management. A scheme for assessing the response to therapy is shown and frequent re-evaluation of disease activity during induction therapy is suggested (Table 3.7); see also *The lupus activity criteria count, LACC*[23]. Cyclo-

TABLE 3.7 Scheme for assessing activity of SLE with nephritis

1. Eliminate infection
2. Eliminate other causes of renal dysfunction, e.g. renal vein thrombosis
3. Evaluate clinical response:
   (a) Severity of extrarenal manifestations (Table 3.1)
   (b) Nephritis: glomerular morphology
   urine deposit: red cell, cast } excretion
   proteinuria
4. Consider relevant serological or immunological factors known to correlate with disease activity in the individual, e.g. rising DNA binding; falling C3, CH50; CRP*; leucopaenia; thrombocytopaenia

SLE is associated with relatively low CRP values when active. *CRP values above 60 mg/L generally indicate superadded infection

phosphamide has a potentially better therapeutic effect than azathioprine from both theoretical and experimental viewpoints, especially when used for the clinical indications outlined. The pooled analysis did not reach such a conclusion – of improved renal survival using cyclophosphamide in patients with diffuse proliferative glomerular nephritis – but there may have been a trend which did not achieve significance[22]. Some physicians are reluctant to consider using cyclophosphamide because of possible mutagenicity[24]. Associations with bladder cancer, however, are found in patients receiving the drug for periods exceeding 5 years[25]. Limited use for 8 weeks, as suggested, is unlikely to confer such risks and the physician must make his own evaluation of its use in individual cases. It is the author's opinion that severe life-threatening lupus with nephritis can be controlled safely in some individuals with short-term cyclophosphamide, where response to other therapy is incomplete.

There is little doubt that acute deterioration in renal function from initially normal GFR as a result of rapidly progressive nephritis merit appropriate steroid and immunosuppressive treatment. With repeated episodes, stepwise loss of renal function is likely with residual renal scarring. Where there is significant pre-existing renal dysfunction, aggressive therapy is less likely to preserve renal function. Patients with pre-existing serum creatinine concentrations in excess of 400 μmol L^{-1} are unlikely to benefit except in control of the disease in organs other than the kidney and perhaps have increased morbidity from the treatment.

Maintenance therapy

The therapeutic aims in the stable patient are to prevent further renal deterioration and to detect and treat exacerbations early. Guidelines for assessing disease activity continue to be relevant (Table 3.7). Therapy will in general be the minimum dose of prednisolone and/or azathioprine to induce a remission. Major unresolved problems remain in the management of this phase. Should azathioprine be withdrawn from the well patient with stable renal function and normal urine deposit? Should steroids be withdrawn in the absence of proteinuria? Such decisions require to be evaluated in the knowledge of the previous behaviour of the individual's disease in response to similar therapeutic manoeuvres. A rational general approach is gradually to reduce steroid dosage, followed by azathioprine to 1 mg kg^{-1}, aiming for withdrawal of therapy at about 2 years. This policy needs to be modified with phasic changes of activity of SLE and re-evaluated frequently. When an individual has previously relapsed on similar reductions in therapy, longer term treatment with azathioprine and low-dose prednisolone may be warranted.

Treatment for renal lesions of lesser severity

The low-grade proliferative forms of glomerulopathies associated with SLE – WHO classes II and III (Table 3.2) – represent 20–50% of the histological grades in series published during the last 15 years. Major dilemmas remain in deciding the best therapy for these patients especially as the severity of their SLE in other organ systems does not usually merit potent immunosuppressive therapy.

Low-grade proliferative glomerulopathies

Although the general conclusions of the pooled analysis[22] do not permit definitive statements on the prognosis of individual renal lesions or on the response to therapy, few would doubt that low-grade proliferative glomerular lesions are capable of producing renal scarring. No significant differences have been detected in the distribution of prognostic factors, chronicity or activity index, in the benefit from appropriate cytotoxic therapy or between individual WHO classes of renal histology[20]. These data suggest that appropriate steroid and immunosuppressive therapy improves long-term outcome in the low-grade proliferative lupus glomerulopathies. Azathioprine is the more appropriate cytotoxic agent for treating this group.

Membranous nephropathy

Lupus membranous nephropathy is reported in 7–26% of lupus glomerulopathies. The lesion is generally considered benign, but a prognosis similar to that of idiopathic membranous disease is reported, with 10–50% showing progressive impairment of renal function[2,14,26]. Comparability with idiopathic membranous nephropathy has also been highlighted in studies in children[27]. Extrarenal manifestations of SLE are common[26]. The association of lupus membranous nephropathy with nephrotic syndrome, often indicates the need for therapy. As with idiopathic membranous disease, there are no well-defined regimens, although the possible benefits of steroids in idiopathic disease have been re-evaluated by the Medical Research Council following completion of a multicentre trial, and a number of other recent controlled studies have shown benefit of cytotoxics, including chlorambucil, in preserving renal function in these patients. Steroid therapy on a trial basis may be warranted for the patient with lupus membraneous nephropathy who is either severely nephrotic or has declining renal function. A suggested regimen is prednisolone, 60 mg/day for up to 4 weeks, 45 mg/day for a further 4 weeks, with frequent review of response. Such therapy can result in gratifying resolution of nephrotic syndrome (Figure 3.2). The frequent coexistence of low- or moderate-grade proliferative changes in the glomeruli of patients with lupus membranous nephropathy suggests that these patients merit additional azathioprine.

Bolus steroids

Short-duration steroid therapy has been used in an attempt to reduce the complications of conventional oral therapy. There are advocates of high-dose 'pulsed' intravenous methylprednisolone[28], escalating dose steroids, and prolonged high-dose oral steroids (e.g. prednisolone, 60 mg/day for 2 months). Proponents cite the capacity of bolus steroids rapidly to improve renal function and reduce peripheral blood lymphocyte counts as evidence for their efficacy. None of the treatment regimens using intravenous bolus doses of steroids have been compared with oral prednisolone in controlled prospective studies which examine benefit and resulting morbidity; choice of therapy is often a matter of a centre's experience and practice. Rapid improvement in extrarenal disease was, however, reported in all of 25 patients with

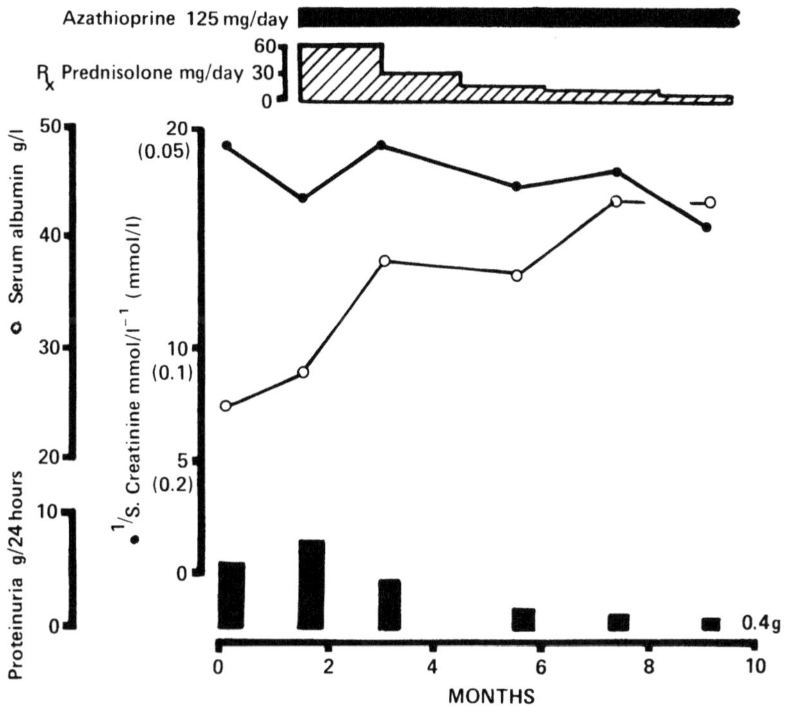

FIGURE 3.2 Resolution of nephrotic syndrome in a female patient with lupus membranous nephropathy following treatment with steroids and azathioprine

diffuse proliferative lupus nephritis given bolus steroids and up to three consecutive courses of methyl prednisolone; 1 g daily for 3 days have been used without significant morbidity[29]. In this series, however, one-third of the patients also received cytotoxic drugs and all received maintenance oral prednisolone, making it difficult to interpret the possible additional benefit of bolus steroids.

Much of the difficulty in evaluating responses to additional bolus steroid therapy lies in the interpretation of the time course of the response to initial induction therapy. Anecdotal reports of benefit are common. One example is shown (Figure 3.3) where a patient with a quantifiable effect of cerebral lupus – deafness – severe diffuse proliferative glomerulonephritis and fever, did not improve following

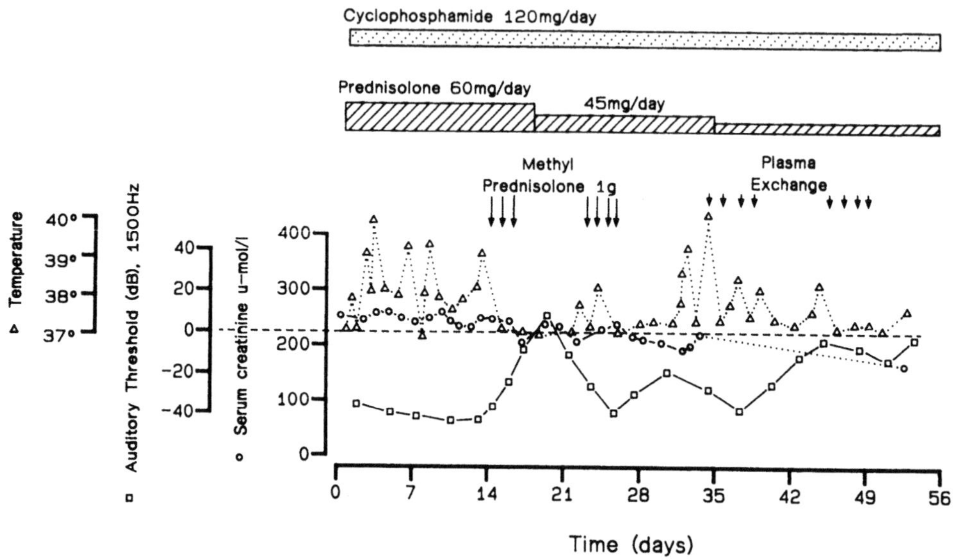

FIGURE 3.3 Anecdotal evidence for benefit of bolus steroids or plasma exchange in a 24-year-old female with cerebral lupus and diffuse proliferative glomerulonephritis: temporary resolution of deafness and fever with each therapeutic manoeuvre

therapy with prednisolone 60 mg/day and cyclophosphamide for two weeks. Fever and deafness responded, albeit temporarily, after each of two courses of additional bolus steroids, followed by plasma exchange. The patient ultimately made a satisfactory recovery.

Plasma exchange

Whilst it is tempting to equate the immediate effects of plasma exchange – reduced circulating DNA-binding capacity, immunoglobulins and immune complexes – with clinical improvement, convincing evidence of benefit has not been established, nor have the circumstances in which it might prove most beneficial. Plasma exchange without the use of cytotoxic therapy in mild systemic lupus without nephritis is ineffective[30] and seems unnecessary. There seems little doubt, however, that there are examples of clinical improvement following plasma exchange in patients with severe lupus nephritis with systemic disease[31-33]. Rapid improvement with abrogation of progressive scarring renal lesions is claimed in uncontrolled studies using plasma exchange with azathioprine or cyclophosphamide[34]. Proof that renal and other system disease improve as a consequence of plasma exchange is subject to the constraints and problems of analysis similar to those outlined for drug therapy of lupus nephritis.

The presence of anticardiolipin antibodies is now firmly established as a risk factor for thrombosis in SLE with or without nephritis. Plasma exchange may be used to remove these antibodies. IgM anticardiolipin antibody which has a predominantly intravascular compartment distribution, is removed almost completely in two 4-litre exchanges, whereas IgG antibodies require more intensive exchanges. Even when a cytotoxic agent is used in combination with plasma exchange, the return of anticardiolipin antibodies is not prevented, although the half-life of re-synthesis and return of detectable levels in serum can be increased from 7 to 14 days (IgM) and from 10 to 20 days (IgG); equilibrium levels of circulating antibody may also be reduced. The therapeutic benefit of this manoeuvre is, however, unproved.

The outstanding question from a nephrological point of view is whether plasma exchange with steroid and cytotoxic drugs confers any advantage over drugs alone in the treatment of the patient with acute resistant lupus nephritis. Such a study can only be approached prospectively on a selective but multicentred basis using as homogeneous a group of patients as possible – for example, those with diffuse proliferative nephritis who have failed to improve after a defined period of drug therapy. Plasma exchange will continue to be regarded as a treatment of final resort for the patient with life-threatening lupus until such answers are available.

Haemostatic abnormalities in lupus nephritis

Thrombocytopaenia and prolonged clotting times can accompany active SLE and may co-exist with thrombotic complications. The mechanism is multifactorial and has been the subject of intense investigation.

Lupus anticoagulant is most often an IgG, occasionally IgM,

autoantibody with affinity for phospholipid fractions of platelets (Factor III). Its presence is suspected when coagulation tests dependent on phospholipid are prolonged (commonly kaolin clotting time and prothrombin time). The abnormality is not corrected by addition of normal plasma unlike clotting factor deficiencies. Explanations of the thrombotic tendency include altered platelet adhesion and interference with vascular prostacyclin formation, or with antithrombin III activity. Thrombosis is a potential complication in all patients with nephrotic syndrome[35], in part due to urinary loss of antithrombin III, as well as abnormal synthesis of coagulation factors. The association of lupus anticoagulant in SLE with recurrent spontaneous abortion, cerebral vessel, venous and intrapulmonary thromboses is well known[36,37].

Patients with lupus nephritis and lupus anticoagulant are particularly predisposed to thrombotic complications. Sixty percent of those with nephrotic-range proteinuria and circulating anticardiolipin antibodies are reported to experience thrombotic events[38]. Administering corticosteroids reduced circulating levels of anticoagulant in 13 of 23 patients treated, in parallel with clinical evidence of disease suppression. No prospective study of such therapy, or of formal anticoagulation, has been undertaken, but either therapeutic manoeuvre should be considered in these particularly high-risk patients. Acute deterioration in renal function in patients with lupus anticoagulant may result from glomerular microvascular thromboses (Figure 3.4) detectable on renal biopsy.

Drug-induced lupus nephritis

Reported associations between drugs and lupus-like disease are increasing. Atenolol, procainamide, isoniazid, quinidine, carbamazepine and others are implicated. The recognition that SLE-like disease, induced by hydralazine, is not uncommon in genetically predisposed individuals[39,40] has been extended to descriptions of segmental proliferative necrotizing and crescentic glomerulonephritis in these patients[41]. The serological markers are characteristic of SLE – both ANF and DNA binding may be present, with hypocomplementaemia or lupus anticoagulant[42]. Those at risk are those

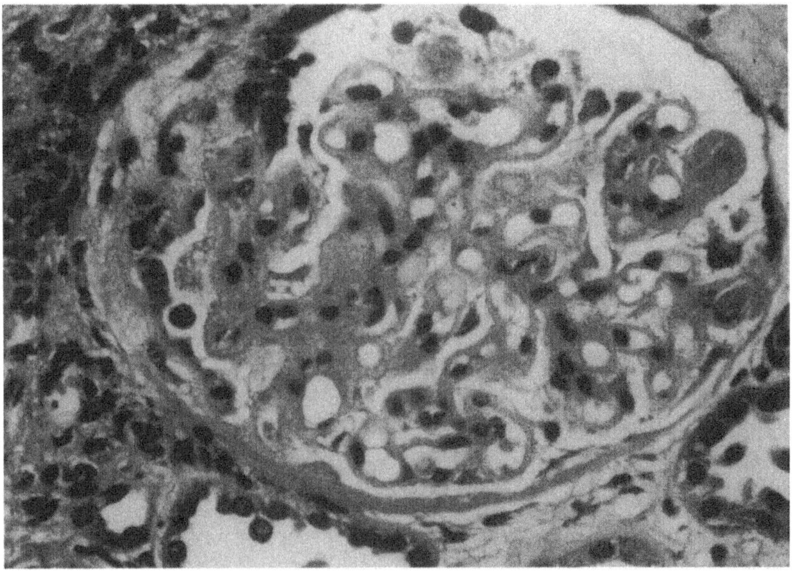

FIGURE 3.4 Intraglomerular thrombosis in a patient with lupus nephritis and circulating anticardiolipin antibody

who are predisposed to hydralazine-associated disease of the milder form – that is, females who are slow acetylators, of tissue type HLA DR4, and who receive a high cumulative dose of the drug. Nephritis is not necessarily accompanied by significant systemic disease and about 50% of the patients respond to withdrawal of the drug. Others may require immunosuppressive therapy[41].

At concentrations equivalent to therapeutic blood levels, hydralazine and isoniazid inhibit *in vitro*[43] the covalent binding of complement component C4b. It is implicit that solubilization of immune complexes by complement is thereby inhibited – a mechanism similar to that proposed in the pathogenesis of idiopathic SLE where patients have complement polymorphism – a null allele[44] for C4a or C4b. These findings are likely to provide only part of the explanation for the induction of lupus nephritis by such drugs as hydralazine, and should be viewed against the broader and newer concepts of the pathogenesis of the disease.

EVOLVING CONCEPTS ON THE PATHOGENESIS OF LUPUS NEPHRITIS

Immunopathogenesis

Since Friou *et al.*'s pioneering work describing the presence of antinuclear factor in the serum of affected patients[45], there has been much experimental work, and many studies in man, on the pathogenesis of SLE. The role of C type retroviruses in murine lupus remains uncertain[46,47] and there is no convincing evidence of a parallel in human disease. Many regard systemic lupus as a breakdown of self-tolerance. Whatever the basis of autoimmunity, SLE is conceptualized as the prototype immune complex disease[48,49]. Circulating immune complexes have in general correlated poorly with the severity or morphology of the glomerular lesions although there are many examples of such associations[50]. This mechanism of induction of nephritis does not provide an explanation for the rarity of recurrence of lupus nephritis in the allografted cadaver kidney. Recurrent lupus nephritis has, however, been reported in a transplant recipient receiving a live related donor graft, which presumably shared intrinsic glomerular antigens with the recipient[51].

Glomerular immune deposits of a granular type found in most lupus nephritides have been frequently regarded as due to trapping of circulating immune complexes. Non-linear immune deposits are now known to result in some nephritides from binding of circulating antibody to fixed discrete glomerular antigens: in an increasing number of nephritides in man, glomerular antoantigens have been described. In animal models of membranous nephropathy – Heymann nephritis – a glycoprotein of molecular weight 330 kDa localized on the glomerular epithelial cell displays the target antigen. The recent observation that monoclonal antibodies to DNA bind to determinants in normal glomerular tissues provides a new initiative into the pathogenesis of glomerular injury in lupus nephritis. It has also recently been shown that, in man, circulating anti-DNA antibodies cross react with antigens in heparan sulphate proteoglycan – a major glycosaminoglycan constituent of glomerular basement membrane and other basement membranes within the body[52]. Inhibition studies indicated the presence of shared antigenic determinants between DNA and heparan sulphate, and serum anti-DNA antibody titres correlated with circulating anti-heparan sulphate titres (Figure 3.5). These findings provide powerful evidence that lupus nephritis might result from *in situ* immune complex formation, analogous to antiglomerular basement membrane disease (Goodpasture's syndrome) and Heymann nephritis. Furthermore,

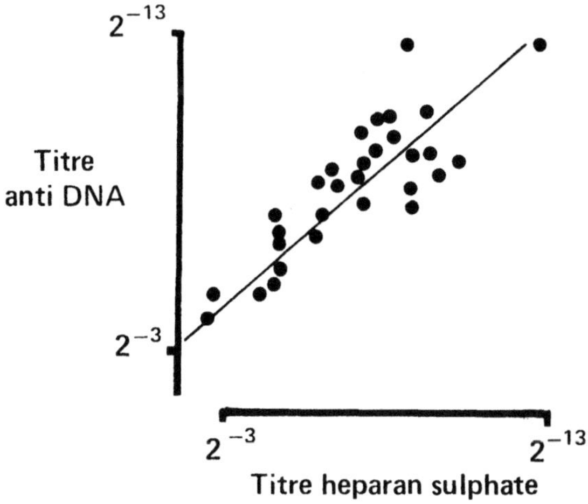

FIGURE 3.5 Correlation between serum anti-DNA antibody and anti-heparan sulphate proteoglycan titres in SLE. (Reproduced from Ref. 52 with permission)

transitions from high to low avidity anti-DNA antibodies can be reflected in transformation in morphology of the glomerular lesion[53]. These changes in affinity, if similarly reflected in variation in autoimmunity to heparan sulphate – intrinsic glomerular antigens – will have important implications in the pathogenesis of the different glomerular lesions of SLE.

Ostensibly, there is considerable diversity of autoantibodies in lupus serum. In addition to characteristic nucleic acid and other cytoplasmic constituent antibodies, autoimmunity is described to a wide range of cell surface antigens and phospholipids. Clinical disease expression with corresponding organ involvement has been described with antibodies to neuronal cells, lymphocyte membranes, vascular endothelium, cardiolipin and the CRI receptor present on several cell types[54,55]. There is evidence that these lupus autoantibodies have restricted diversity[56] and that an epitope is shared between target antigens on different cell types in SLE. The epitope may originate in the phosphodiester-bonded structures of DNA nucleotide and is common to DNA, cardiolipin and a circulating procoagulant protein[57]. These findings suggest that B cell activation in SLE might involve a restricted population only. The significance of restricted idiotype diversity in the pathogenesis of lupus nephritis remains to be elucidated. Cross-reactive anti-idiotypic antibodies, when administered to the lupus-prone mouse, significantly reduce nephritis and prolong survival[58]. Glomerular antigens containing heparan sulphate are potentially cross reactive with restricted diversity autoantibodies in SLE, and this has important conceptual and therapeutic implications in future approaches to investigation of the pathogenesis of lupus nephritis in man.

Immunological evaluation

Systemic lupus is characterized by diverse abnormalities of the immune system. The uncertainty surrounding the precise mechanism by which end-organ injury is mediated reflects the problems of defining reliable indices of disease activity. There is still doubt that serological or other markers tell the clinician more than observation and renal biopsy.

The serological and cellular abnormalities detected in SLE express the associated immunoregulatory abnormalities, and have been adequately reviewed[59]. Longitudinal studies have shown that no single test is of value in defining disease activity as a discriminant for alteration of a clinical feature[60]. On categorizing all SLE patients into those with nephritis, cerebritis, arthralgias and cutaneous vasculitis, no single test was found to distinguish the groups reliably. The tests were found to differ in their ability to reflect disease activity when these subgroups were analysed. Several studies have described the level of circulating IgG anti-ds- (double stranded-) DNA antibodies of high avidity and which fix complement as markers of the severity of nephritis. Others claim IgM, anti-ds-DNA to be of significance. Severely active nephritis, in general, is usually accompanied by high ds-DNA binding, often with low C3 and C4[9,60]. More subtle changes of lymphopaenia and thrombocytopaenia should not be overlooked[60].

The lack of consistency between the published studies evaluating clinicopathological correlants is, in part, explained by study design. In a long-term prospective study of 143 patients with SLE, 33 developed evidence of active SLE. Twenty-one of these had nephritis or deteriorations in pre-existing renal disease[61]. A rising anti-ds-DNA antibody preceded flares in each patient, with a doubling time of titre of 6 weeks in most, but the actual exacerbations were characterized by a rapidly decreasing antibody level. Decreasing C4 levels, then C1q and C3 accompany the early phase and flare. Changes in the titres of serological indices for an individual patient may be of greater value than absolute levels and can provide useful reassurance for the clinician that a new clinical feature may be a consequence of SLE.

MORTALITY

The causes of mortality in patients with lupus nephritis are similar to those of all patients with SLE. Early deaths are the result of active lupus or intercurrent infection, with late deaths occurring from cardiovascular disease[62]. This bimodal pattern has been observed in other studies[63]. Mortality in the early phase reflects the difficulties in balancing the suppression of kidney and other organ involvement of SLE, whilst minimizing risks of infection from therapy – especially in the patient with advancing uraemia. Vascular disease is a result of accelerated atheroma in 50% of patients dying from SLE under the age of 40 and appears to be associated with SLE of longer duration[62], hypertension, hyperlipidaemia and lupus carditis, rather than steroid dosage[64]. Lupus vasculitis of the coronary vessels is also reported and can affect children[63]. It is likely that the presence of lupus anticoagulant exacerbates the tendency to occlusive arterial disease[65,66].

A reduction in nephritis-related deaths was found in the pooled analysis when combined cytotoxic and steroid therapy was compared with prednisolone alone[22]. Near significance values were revealed in comparisons of all deaths (Table 3.6). Patients receiving azathioprine or cyclophosphamide require significantly less prednisolone when steroid dosage is tailored to individual needs and fewer steroid complications occur[22]. It is tempting to attribute reduced mortality to such a steroid-sparing effect.

In a major analysis of infection and immunosuppression in immunologically-mediated disease, higher-dose steroids used in patients with impaired renal function proved to be a high risk factor for serious infective complications[67]. Cyclophosphamide was associated with infection only in the presence of neutropaenia and the duration of plasma exchange was unrelated to frequency of infection. Bacteria accounted for the majority of infections. Serious opportunist pathogens, however, accounted for 14% of infections in patients with lupus nephritis[67]. These findings further support the broad conclusions of the pooled analysis that appropriate and careful use of cytotoxic therapy, whilst minimizing steroid dose in lupus nephritis, can reduce morbidity and mortality.

Patients who reach end-stage renal failure but who require therapy for control of SLE involving organs other than the kidneys may be particularly susceptible to steroid-induced mortality[68]. Management of the lupus patient in end-stage renal failure is as difficult as in other phases of the disease. Survival of patients undergoing long-term dialysis is comparable to that of the general dialysis population[69,70]. Patients with acute deterioration in renal function prior to dialysis are more likely to have continuing disease activity and higher mortality than those with slowly progressive renal failure[70]. In those surviving, clinical and serological evidence of lupus activity tends to abate[68,69], allowing reduction in immunosuppressive therapy. A general approach to the lupus patient receiving maintenance dialysis – to adjust treatment meticulously to requirements – is as important as in other phases of disease. Recovery of renal function continues to be documented in a significant minority. The absence of active SLE as well as the rarity of recurrence of nephritis in those patients receiving allografts may have pathogenetic implications discussed previously, but, as yet, remains unexplained.

Major problems persist in the management of lupus nephritis. Our incomplete understanding of its pathogenesis makes it difficult to identify any manoeuvre which will improve prognosis or reduce complications. Although important advances have been made in our knowledge of the immunopathogenesis of B cell hyperactivity apparent in systemic lupus, and in the genetic and hormonal modulation of the severity of disease, the underlying mechanism of autoimmunity and consequent nephritis remains unknown. The restricted diversity of lupus autoantibodies suggests that specific treatment of lupus nephritis may be possible by idiotype manipulation. Further understanding of the pathogenetic function involved will allow us to design relevant immunotherapeutic strategies in our future approaches to this disease.

REFERENCES

1. Tan, E. M., Cohen, A. S. and Fries, J. F. (1982). The 1982 revised criteria for the classification of systemic lupus erythematosus. *Arthritis Rheum.*, **25,** 11, 1271–1277
2. Baldwin, D. S., Gluck, M. C. and Lowenstein, J. (1977). Lupus nephritis: Clinical course as related to morphologic forms and their transitions. *Am. J. Med.*, **62,** 12–30
3. Leehey, D. J., Katz, A. I. and Azaran, A. H. (1982). Silent diffuse lupus nephritis: long term follow up. *Am. J. Kidney Dis.*, **2,** (Suppl. 1), 188–196
4. Bennett, W. M., Bardana, E. J. and Houghton, D. C. (1977). Silent renal involvement in systemic lupus erythematosus. *Int. Arch. Allergy Appl. Immunol.*, **55,** 420–428
5. Terai, C., Nojima, K. and Takano, A. (1987). Determination of urinary albumin excretion by radioimmunoassay in patients with subclinical lupus nephritis. *Clin. Nephrol.*, **27,** 2, 79–83
6. Adu, D., Williams, D. G. and Taube, D. (1983). Late onset systemic lupus erythematosus and Lupus-like disease in patients with apparent idiopathic glomerulonephritis. *Q. J. Med.*, **208,** 471–487
7. Appel, G. B., Silva, F. G. and Pirani, C. L. (1978). Renal involvement in systemic lupus erythematosus. A study of 56 patients. *Medicine*, **57,** 371–410
8. Cameron, J. S., Turner, D. R. and Ogg, C. S. (1979). Systemic lupus with nephritis: a long-term study. *Q. J. Med.*, **189,** 1–24
9. Miller, M. H., Urowitz, M. B. and Gladman, D. D. (1983). Systemic lupus in males. *Medicine*, **62,** 5, 327–333
10. Yeung, C. K., Ng, W. L. and Wong, W. S. (1985). Acute deteriorations in renal function in systemic lupus erythematosus. *Q. J. Med.*, **219,** 393–402
11. Ropes, M. W. (1964). Observations on the natural course of disseminated lupus erythematosus. *Medicine*, **43,** 387–391
12. Hecht, B., Siegel, N. and Adler, S. (1976). Prognostic indices in lupus nephritis. *Medicine*, **55,** 2, 163–181
13. Donadio, J. V., Burgess, J. H. and Holley, K. E. (1977). Membranous lupus nephropathy: a clinicopathological study. *Medicine*, **56,** 6, 527–536
14. Banfi, G., Mazzucco, G. and Di Belgiojoso, G. B. (1985). Morphological parameters in lupus nephritis: their relevance for classification and relationship with clinical and histological findings and outcome. *Q. J. Med.*, **217,** 153–168
15. Tateno, S., Kobayashi, Y. and Hidekazu, S. (1983). Study of lupus nephritis: its classification and the significance of subendothelial deposits. *Q. J. Med.*, **207,** 311–331
16. Donadio, J. V. (1984). Cytotoxic drug treatment of lupus nephritis. *N. Engl. J. Med.*, **311,** 8, 528–529

17. Austin, H. A., Muenz, L. R. and Joyce, K. M. (1984). Diffuse proliferative lupus nephritis: identification of specific pathological features affecting renal outcome. *Kidney Int.*, **25,** 689–695
18. Magil, A. B., Ballon, H. S. and Chan, V. (1984). Diffuse proliferative lupus glomerulonephritis. *Medicine,* **63,** 4, 210–220
19. Glassock, R. J., Cohen, A. H. and Adler, S. G. (1986). Secondary glomerular diseases. In Brenner and Rector (eds.) *The Kidney*, 3rd Edn. (Philadelphia: W. B. Saunders)
20. Balow, J. E., Austin, H. A. and Muenz, L. R. (1984). Effect of treatment on the evolution of renal abnormalities in lupus nephritis. *N. Engl. J. Med.,* **311,** 8, 491–495
21. Wagner, L. (1976). Immunosuppressive agents in lupus nephritis: a critical analysis. *Medicine,* **55,** 3, 239–250
22. Felson, D. T. and Anderson, J. (1984). Evidence for superiority of immunosuppressive drugs and prednisone over prednisone alone in lupus nephritis. *N. Engl. J. Med.,* **311,** 24, 1528–1533
23. Urowitz, M. B., Gladman, D. D. and Tozman, E. C. (1984). The lupus activity criteria count (LACC). *J. Rheumatol.*, **11,** 783–787
24. Kinlen, L. J., Sheil, A. G. R. and Peto, J. (1979). Collaborative United Kingdom–Australasian study of cancer in patients treated with immunosuppressive drugs. *Br. Med. J.,* **2,** 1461–1416
25. Elliott, R. W., Essenhigh, D. M. and Morley, A. R. (1982). Cyclosphosphamide treatment of systemic lupus erythematosus: risk of bladder cancer exceeds benefit. *Br. Med. J.,* **284,** 1160–1161
26. Gonzalez-Dettoni, H. and Tron, F. (1985). Membranous glomerulopathy in SLE. *Adv. Nephrol.,* **14,** 347–364
27. The Southwest Paediatric Nephrology Study Group (1986). Comparisons of idiopathic and lupus membranous nephropathy in children. *Am. J. Kidney Dis.*, **7** (2), 115–124
28. Kimberley, R. P., Lockshin, M. D. and Sherman, R. L. (1981). High dose intravenous methylprednisolone pulse therapy in systemic lupus erythematosus. *Am. J. Med.,* **70,** 817–824
29. Ponticelli, C., Zucchelli, P. and Banfi, G. (1982). Treatment of diffuse proliferative lupus nephritis by intravenous high dose methyl prednisolone. *Q. J. Med.,* **201,** 16–24
30. Wei, N., Klippel, J. H. and Huston, D. P. (1983). Randomised trial of plasma exchange in mild systemic lupus erythematosus. *Lancet,* **1,** 17–21
31. Verrier Jones, J., Cumming, R. H. and Bucknall, R. C. (1976). Plasmapheresis in the management of acute systemic lupus erythematosus. *Lancet,* **1,** 709–711
32. Lockwood, C. M., Rees, A. J. and Russell, B. (1977). Experience of the use of plasma exchange in the management of potentially fulminating glomerulonephritis and SLE. *Exp. Haemtol.,* **5,** 117–136
33. Verrier Jones, J., Cumming, R. H. and Bacon, P. A. (1979). Evidence for a therapeutic effect of plasmapheresis in patients with systemic lupus erythematosus. *Q. J. Med.,* **48,** 555–576
34. Leaher, B. R., Becker, G. J. and Dowliner, J. P. (1986). Rapid improvement in severe lupus glomerular lesions following intensive plasma exchange associated with immunosuppression. *Clin. Nephrol.,* **25,** (5), 236–244

35. Llach, F. (1985). Hypercoagulability, renal vein thrombosis, and other thrombotic complications of nephrotic syndrome. *Kidney Int.*, **28,** 429–439
36. Hughes, G. R. V. (1983). Thrombosis, abortion, cerebral disease and the lupus anticoagulant. *Br. Med. J.*, **287,** 1088–1089
37. Editorial (1984). Lupus anticoagulant. *Lancet,* **1,** 1157–1158
38. Jungers, P., Liote, F. and Dautzenberg, M. D. (1984). Lupus anticoagulant and thrombosis in systemic lupus erythematosus. *Lancet,* **1,** 574–575
39. Mansilla-Tinoco, R., Harland, S. J. and Ryan, P. J. (1982). Hydralazine, antinuclear antibodies, and the lupus syndrome. *Br. Med. J.*, **284**, 936–939
40. Batchelor, J. R., Welsh, K. I. and Mansilla-Tinoco, R. (1980). Hydralazine induced systemic lupus erythematosus: influence of HLA-DR and sex on susceptibility. *Lancet,* **1,** 1107–1109
41. Bjorck, S., Westberg, G. and Svalander, C. (1983). Rapidly progressive glomerulonephritis after hydralazine, *Lancet,* **2,** 42
42. Kincaid Smith, P. and Whitworth, J. A. (1983). Hydralazine-associated glomerulonephritis. *Lancet,* **2,** 348
43. Sim, E., Gill, E. W. and Sim, R. B. (1984). Drugs that induce systemic lupus erythematosus inhibit complement component C4. *Lancet,* **2,** 422–424
44. Fielder, A. H. L., Walport, M. J. and Batchelor, J. R. (1983). Family study of the major histocompatibility complex in patients with systemic lupus erythematosus: importance of null alleles of C4a and C4b. *Br. Med. J.*, **286,** 425–428
45. Friou, G. J., Finch, S. C. and Detri, K. D. (1958). Interaction of nuclei with globulin from lupus erythematosus serum demonstrated with fluorescent antibody. *J. Immunol.*, **80,** 324–329
46. Datta, S. K., Manny, N. and Andrzejewski, C. (1978). Genetic studies of autoimmunity and retrovirus expression in crosses of New Zealand black mice. *J. Exp. Med.*, **147,** 854–871
47. Boumpas, D. T., Popovic, M. and Mann, D. L. (1986). Type C retrovirus of human T cell leukaemia family are not evident in patients with systemic lupus erythematosus. *Arth. Rheum.*, **29,** (2), 185–188
48. Koffler, D., Agnello, V. and Thoburn, R. (1971). Systemic lupus erythematosus: prototype of immune complex nephritis in man. *J. Exp. Med.*, **134,** 3, 169–179
49. Glassock, R. J. (1981). Glomerulonephritis in systemic lupus erythematosus. *Am. J. Nephrol.*, **1,** 53
50. Abrass, C. K., Neis, J. M. and Louie, J. S. (1980). Correlation and predictive accuracy of circulating immune complexes with disease activity in patients with SLE. *Arthritis Rheum.*, **23,** 3, 273–282
51. Kumano, K., Sakai, T. and Mashimo, S. (1987). A case of recurrent lupus nephritis after renal transplantation. *Clin. Nephrol.*, **27,** 2, 94–98
52. Faaber, P., Rijke, T. P. M. and van der Putte, L. B. A. (1986). Cross-reactivity of human and murine anti-DNA antibodies with heparan sulphate. *J. Clin. Invest.*, **77,** 1824–1830
53. Asano, Y. and Nakamoto. Y. (1978). Avidity of anti-DNA antibody and glomerular immune complex localisation in lupus nephritis. *Clin. Nephrol.*, 134–139
54. Cook, J. M., Kazatchkine, M. D. and Bourgeois, P. (1986). Anti C3b-receptor antibodies in patients with SLE. *Clin. Immunol. Immunopathol.*, **38,** 1, 135–138
55. Jacob, L., Lety, M. A. and Bach, J. F. (1986). Human systemic lupus erythematosus sera contain antibodies against cell surface proteins that share epitopes with DNA. *Proc. Natl. Acad. Sci. USA,* **83,** (18), 6970–6974

56. Schwartz, R. S. (1983). Monoclonal lupus autoantibodies. *Immunol. Today*, **4**, 3, 68–69
57. Lafer, E. M., Rauch, J. and Andrzejewski, C. (1981). Polyspecific monoclonal lupus autoantibodies reactive with both polynucleotides and phospholipids. *J. Exp. Med.*, **153**, 897–909
58. Hahn, B. and Ebling, F. (1984). Suppression of murine lupus nephritis by administration of an anti-idiotypic antibody to anti-DNA. *J. Immunol.*, **132**, 187–190
59. Morrow, W. J. W., Youinou, P. and Isenberg, D. A. (1983). Systemic lupus erythematosus: 25 years of treatment related to immunopathology. *Lancet*, **1**, 206–210
60. Morrow, W. J. W., Isenberg, D. A. and Todd-Pokropek, A. (1982). Useful laboratory measurements in the management of systemic lupus erythematosus. *Q. J. Med.*, **51**, 125–138
61. Swaak, A. J. G., Groenwold, J. and Bronsweld, W. (1986). Predictive value of complement profiles and anti-ds DNA in systemic lupus erythematosus. *Ann. Rheum. Dis.*, **45**, 359–366
62. Rubin, L. A., Urowitz, M. B. and Gladman, D. D. (1985). Mortality in systemic lupus erythematosus: the bimodal pattern revisited. *Q. J. Med.*, **216**, 55, 87–98
63. Correia, P., Cameron, J. S. and Lian, J. D. (1985). Why do patients with lupus nephritis die? *Br. Med. J.*, **290**, 126–131
64. Haider, Y. S. and Roberts, W. C. (1981). Coronary arterial disease in systemic lupus erythematosus. *Am. J. Med.*, **70**, 775–781
65. Harris, E. N., Gharavi, A. E. and Boey, M. L. (1983). Anticardiolipin antibodies: detection by radioimmunoassay and association with thrombosis in systemic lupus erythematosus. *Lancet*, **2**, 1211–1214
66. Jungers, P., Liote, F. and Dautzenberg, M. D. (1984). Lupus anticoagulant and thrombosis in systemic lupus erythematosus. *Lancet*, **1**, 574–575
67. Cohen, J., Pinching, A. J. and Rees, A. J. (1982). Infection and immunosuppression. *Q. J. Med.*, **201**, 1–15
68. Coplon, N. S., Diskin, C. J. and Petersen, J. (1983). The long-term clinical course of systemic lupus erythematosus in end-stage renal disease. *N. Engl. J. Med.*, **308**, 4, 186–190
69. Cheigh, J. S., Stenzel, K. H. and Rubin, A. L. (1983). Systemic lupus erythematosus in patients with chronic renal failure. *Am. J. Med.*, **75**, 602–606
70. Correia, P., Cameron, J. S. and Oggk, C. S. (1984). End stage renal failure in systemic lupus erythematosus with nephritis. *Clin. Nephrol.*, **22**, 6, 293–302

4

HENOCH–SCHÖNLEIN DISEASE

R. S. TROMPETER

HISTORICAL NOTE

Schönlein is usually credited with the original description of a characteristic purpuric rash and arthralgia[1], and Henoch with the association of a smiliar rash with abdominal symptoms[2] and subsequently with renal disease[3]. However, as early as 1801, Heberden had described repeated attacks of purpuric rashes with painful swelling, abdominal discomfort and haematuria[4].

> 'Another boy, five years old, was seized with pains and swellings in various parts, and the penis in particular was so distended, though not discoloured, that he could hardly make water. He had sometimes pains in his belly, with vomiting, and at the time some streaks of blood were perceived in his stools, and the urine was tinged with blood. When the pain attacked his leg, he was unable to walk; and presently the skin of his leg was all over full of bloody points. After a truce of three or four days the swelling returned, and the bloody dots, as before'

DEFINITION

The clinical manifestations are legion, but most characteristic are a typical rash, fever, arthritis, gastrointestinal symptoms and renal disease. In its usual form, Henoch–Schönlein purpura (HSP) is a disease of childhood and most patients recover completely within a month of the onset of the initial symptom.

EPIDEMIOLOGY

Most patients are caucasian or oriental, and contributions to the literature during the past decade give the impression that the condition is more common in Europe and Japan than in America. This is also reflected by the numbers of patients entered into a therapeutic trial conducted by the International Study of Kidney Disease in Children (ISKDC) by January, 1980 (Table 4.1).

TABLE 4.1 Geographical distribution of HS nephritis (ISKDC, January, 1980)

Zone	*Centres*	*Patients*
United Kingdom	3	35
Rest of Europe	4	18
North America	6	20
Mexico	1	1

HSP mainly affects children between the ages of 3 and 10 years[5,6]. In decreasing order of incidence, it also occurs in children older than 10 years, babies, adolescents and adults. Boys are affected more often (1.5:1) than girls. In about two-thirds of children, an upper respiratory tract infection precedes the onset of HSP by 1–3 weeks[6]. The incidence shows a seasonal variation with a peak around November to January in the northern hemisphere[8]. In general, children are ill and pyrexial with a temperature usually not higher than 38°C.

PATHOGENESIS

The aetiology is unknown. At the beginning of this century, Osler likened the condition to serum sickness and other anaphylactoid reactions[9]. The term 'anaphylactoid purpura' was introduced by Frank[10]. Since then, the idea that HSP is caused by hypersensitivity reaction has developed into the concept that HSP is caused by an allergy to antigens derived from micro-organisms, food or drugs[11]. Gairdner[12] reported on the high incidence of sore throat and positive cultures of haemolytic streptococci preceding the initial onset or relapses of HSP. His patients or their relatives did not have a higher incidence of allergies, such as asthma, hay fever, or eczema, than control patients. Others have reported a higher incidence of upper respiratory tract infections preceding HSP[7,13]. However, Ayoub and Hoyer[14] were able to show by a carefully controlled study that patients with HSP do not have an increased frequency of positive cultures for haemolytic streptococci. In the majority of HSP cases, an antecedent infection cannot be identified. Various micro-organisms have been implicated in individual cases, including varicella[15], vaccinia[16], rubella[13], measles[13], influenza virus[17] and mycoplasma[18,19].

Allergies to food and drugs have also been incriminated in the pathogenesis of HSP. The intake of dairy products, eggs, chocolate, wheat, and beans have been connected with the development of HSP[11]. Only in a few cases was it shown that repeated intake of a particular kind of food provoked the disease.

A variety of drugs have been implicated in the pathogenesis of HSP, including penicillin, sulphonamides, tetracycline, erythromycin, quinidine, phenacetin, phenothiazines and griseofulvin[20]. However, several of these drugs have been readministered after admission to hospital without exacerbation or recurrence of the disease[7]. Although it cannot be excluded that drugs are involved in the pathogenesis of HSP, evidence fails to support this hypothesis. HSP has also been reported in adults to be associated with carcinoma of the gastro-intestinal and respiratory tract[21,22].

CLINICAL MANIFESTATIONS

Skin

The characteristic rash is purpuric and is symmetrically distributed over the extensor surfaces of the lower legs and arms and over the sides of the buttocks. It is nearly always present in the area of the lateral malleolus and, at times, is present only there. Pressure areas, for example, beneath a waist band, are commonly affected, and a few spots may be present on the penis. It usually begins as a red maculo-papular rash that then becomes purpuric and eventually takes on a fawn colour as it fades. The patches of purpura may be tiny or very large. Sometimes the rash does not have a purpuric stage. It does not itch. In children under 5 years of age, the illness may start with a generalized urticarial rash, which later may become purpuric. Oedema of the scalp and face and of the dorsa of the hands and feet is common. The oedema correlates with the activity of the vasculitis and not with the degree of proteinuria. It has also been attributed to the enteric loss of protein[23]. Subcutaneous bleeding may occur anywhere. It is often seen in the scrotum (mimicking torsion of the testicle), eyelids and conjunctiva.

Joints

The joints are involved in up to 75% of cases. The arthralgia most commonly affects the knees and ankles and, less often, the wrists and fingers. The joints may be painful and swollen because of periarticular oedema. Joint effusions are rare and the arthralgia recovers without leaving residual damage.

Gastrointestinal tract

Colicky abdominal pain is common and may be sufficiently severe to mimic an acute abdominal emergency. Vomiting and diarrhoea are also common and may be accompanied by haematemesis and melaena. Alimentary problems can be most severe, occur in up to 50% of cases, and may precede the joint and skin manifestations. Petechiae and ecchymoses have been observed endoscopically in the stomach, duodenum, sigmoid colon and rectum[24]. Radiologically, the jejunum and ileum are most frequently affected. The local oedema and intramural haemorrhages may appear like thumb prints or pseudotumours[25]. These lesions may occasionally lead to massive gastrointestinal haemorrhage or intussusception.

Kidney

Renal manifestations are found in 20–100% of patients with HSP[7,26,27], and tend to be more common and more severe in older children[7,26]. The reported variable incidence of renal involvement stems from the differing criteria used to define renal involvement as well as by different methods used to detect microscopic haematuria. In 80% of patients with the nephropathy, urinary abnormalities follow the onset of the typical rash within 1 month, and, in most others, occur within 3 months[26]. Occasionally, urinary abnormalities may precede the onset of the rash or follow it by many months. In older patients, severe alimentary system involvement[7,13], frequent relapses of skin lesions[7] and late clinical relapses of skin lesions beyond 3 months[13], have been particularly associated with an increased incidence of renal involvement.

At presentation, microscopic haematuria, with or without proteinuria, occurs in 70–80% of cases of HSP nephropathy, while 20–30% will have gross haematuria. Variable amounts of protein are commonly present, even in urine which does not contain gross blood, and the patient may have nephrotic syndrome. Uraemia, often transient, is found in approximately 20% of children with HSP nephropathy. Hypertension is an uncommon initial feature. A mild focal glomerulonephritis has, however, been reported by independent observers in biopsy specimens obtained from children without clinical evidence of nephritis[13,28].

There is a small, but significant, death rate from renal failure: 3–7.7% of children entering dialysis programmes in Europe[8,29] were suffering from HSP. Counahan *et al.*[30] reported that 14% of a group of 88 children followed up for a mean of 10 years had died or were in chronic renal failure (CRF), while a further 10% had active disease. Their patients were however, mostly selected on the basis of comparatively severe illness clinically, and the mortality rate is an overestimate. In a large Japanese series[31], 123 out of 203 (60.6%) children with HSP showed renal involvement and the estimated death rate of the latter, allowing for 10 children lost to follow-up, was 8.9%.

In the past decade, prediction of the outcome has been the focus of a good deal of attention. Good prognostic criteria are needed because treatment with cytotoxic drugs is, at best, of dubious value[13,29,30], and it is therefore desirable to elaborate a means of detecting those patients who are most greatly at risk, and in whom exposure to the potential hazards of these drugs is justified. For several years, the ISKDC has been conducting a controlled trial in which a course of cyclophosphamide given for six weeks is compared with supportive treatment only. The number of patients who have satisfied the trial criteria and have been followed up for 2 years is, however, as yet too small to yield meaningful results.

A clinical presentation with a mixed nephritic–nephrotic pattern has, for many years, been recognized as denoting a poor prognosis[13,29,30]. Even so, 47–54% of these patients were either in complete remission or had only minor urinary abnormalities an average of 6–10 years after onset[30,32]. Counahan *et al.*[30] extended the minimum observation period of the patients originally reported by Meadow *et al.*[13] from 2 to 6½ years and noted that the proportion of patients who had either died, were in chronic renal failure, or showed active disease had increased from 20–24%. A disturbing feature was that 4 children with a non-nephritic clinical presentation were doing badly: one had died, one was on regular dialysis and two were in early CRF. Thus, the clinical presentation is not a very good discriminator of prognosis.

HISTOPATHOLOGY

Light microscopy

Few post-mortem studies of fatal cases of HSP have been reported. Most of the histological documentation has been obtained from skin and kidney biopsies. The lesion most typical of HSP consists of a leucoblastic vasculitis, which is characterized by a transmural and perivascular infiltration with polymorphonuclear leuocytes, histiocytes, and sometimes eosinophils in association with fibrinoid necrosis, nuclear debris, and extravasation of erythrocytes. This lesion is frequently found in the superficial postcapillary venules of the skin. The involvement of a high percentage of glomeruli with epithelial crescents is claimed to denote a bad prognosis[29,30,32] (Figure 4.1). The problem of defining crescents and quantitating them with accuracy is a considerable one, leading to over or under estimation of size of crescents or the number of glomeruli affected. The group of patients in whom prognostication is paticularly hazardous are those with 50–75% crescentic glomeruli; about 60% of those patients appear to do well[30,32].

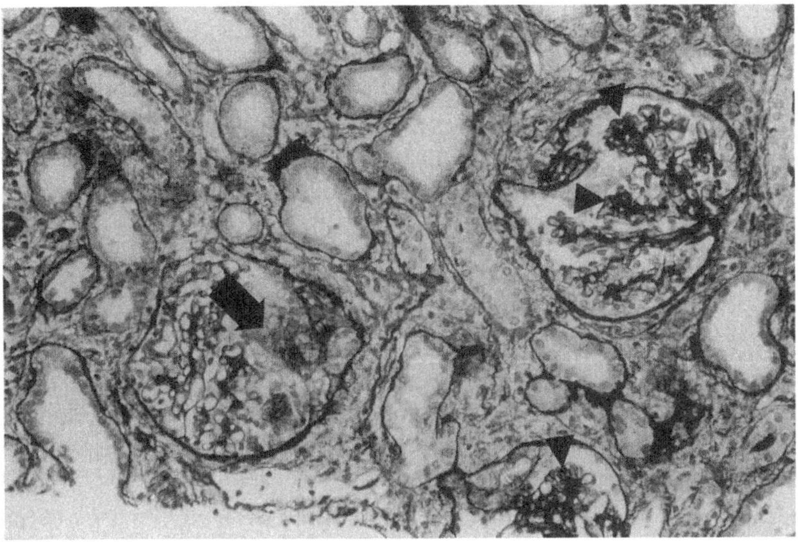

FIGURE 4.1 One of the 3 glomeruli present has a cellular crescent (arrow). The other two show increase in mesangial matrix and some collapse of loops (arrow head). Mesangial cell proliferation is also present but not obvious on this preparation (silver impregnation × 170)

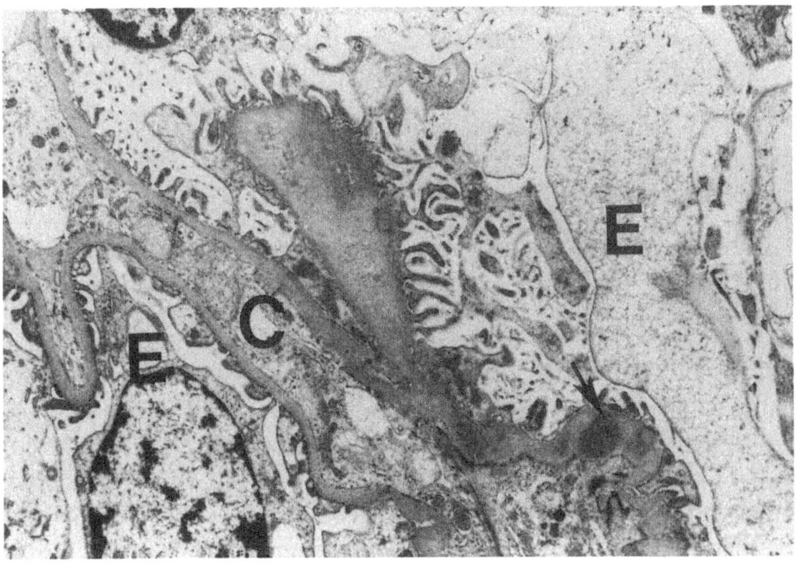

FIGURE 4.2 This glomerular capillary loop (C) is collapsed and intramembranous deposits are present (arrow). Epithelial cells (E) are swollen and there is focal foot process effacement. (Photoelectronmicrograph × 3700)

Immunofluorescence

The immunoflourescence pattern of HS nephritis is predominantly diffuse mesangial IgA, often with less deposits of other immunoglobulins and complement components, especially C3. Capillary wall deposits are sometimes observed, particularly in those cases with extensive crescent formation[8].

Electron microscopy

Electron-dense deposits are predominantly mesangial but are also seen in subendothelial and subepithelial locations, the latter somewhat less frequently[8,32] (Figure 4.2).

According to the system used by Counahan *et al.*[30], patients may be considered in terms of four clinical states:

State A – Normal: physical examination (including blood pressure), urine and GFR all normal;

State B – Minor urinary abnormalities: normal physical examination and GFR, with microscopic haematuria or proteinuria $<40\,\mathrm{mg\,h^{-1}\,m^{-2}}$ ($<1.0\,\mathrm{g\,(24\,h)^{-1}}$);

State C – Active renal disease: proteinuria $\geqslant 40\,\mathrm{mg\,h^{-1}\,m^{-1}}$ ($\geqslant 1\,\mathrm{g\,(24\,h)^{-1}}$) or hypertension (diastolic BP persistently $\geqslant 90$ mmHg) or both, with GFR $60\,\mathrm{ml\,min^{-1}\,(1.73\,m^2)^{-1}}$;

State D – Renal insufficiency: active renal disease but with GFR $60\,\mathrm{ml\,min^{-1}\,(1.73\,m^2)^{-1}}$ (including dialysis and transplantation) or deceased.

A group of patients was followed for a mean observation period of 6 years. Table 4.2 shows the results in 50 children with adequate tissue available for EM examination. It can be seen that all 6 children in state D and 3 out of 5 in state C showed subepithelial deposits associated with subendothelial and mesangial deposits. Heaton *et al.*[33] noted that subepithelial deposits were generally seen where the light microscopy changes were more severe; the authors, however, did not discuss the relationship of these histological features to outcome.

TABLE 4.2 Relationship between location of deposits on EM and outcome[32]

		Follow-up status			
Location of deposits	*n*	*A*	*B*	*C*	*D*
None	1	—	1	—	—
Mesangial only	16	9	6	1	—
Mesangial + subendothelial	17	12	4	1	—
Mesangial + subepithelial	1	1	—	—	—
All 3 locations	15	3	3	3	6

LABORATORY INVESTIGATIONS

To date, no laboratory test has been found to be diagnostic for HSP. The peripheral blood count may show neutrophil leukocytosis. The erythrocyte sedimentation rate can be elevated. Platelet count, bleeding time and clotting time are normal. Positive throat cultures and elevated ASO, anti-DNase, and anti-NADase titres have no diagnostic significance. Tests for antinuclear antibodies and rheumatoid factor are negative.

Serum IgA levels may be transiently elevated in approximately 50% of children with HSP[34]. About half of the children with HSP have cryoglobulins in their sera: IgA and properdin were detected in these cryoglobulins[35]. These findings suggest that cryoglobulins containing IgA can activate the alternative pathway. Although complement levels are consistently normal in HSP, C3d levels are significantly elevated in the acute phase of HSP as an expression of a higher turn over of C3, possibly by activation via the alternative pathway. The finding of deposits of IgA, C3 and C5 in cutaneous vessel walls in the absence of C1q and C4 would support this hypothesis.

Several groups of investigators have demonstrated the presence of IgA-containing immune complexes in patients with HSP[36–38]. The immunological abnormalities are transient and tend to return to normal as the acute phase of the illness subsides.

The glomerular mesangial deposition of IgA, IgG and C3 in HSP nephropathy suggests that the renal lesions in the disease result from the deposition of immune complexes. *In situ* immune-complex formation, with IgA circulating as an antibody against mesangial antigens, seems unlikely to be a cause of the lesions because it does not explain the systemic manifestations and the common presence of IgA-containing deposits in cutaneous vessels[39] and the intestine in the disease. More likely, HSP nephropathy results from circulating soluble immune complexes having characteristics that permit their generalized small-vessel and renal mesangial deposition. Circulating IgA-containing immune complexes[38,39] have been found early in the course of the disease, during stages of active vasculitis, in a large proportion of patients with HSP, further suggesting their role in the pathogenesis of the disease.

TREATMENT

There is no evidence from adequately controlled studies that any specific treatment affects the course of either Henoch–Schönlein syndrome or the associated nephritis. There are many anecdotal reports of diminution of gastrointestinal symptoms with corticosteroid therapy[7]. Corticosteroids may have also been given for the renal disease; analysis of retrospective data does not show a definite benefit[13]. Immunosuppressive drugs have been used, including azathioprine, cyclophosphamide, and combinations of corticosteroids, cyclophosphamide, dipyridamole and oral anticoagulants.

Although many spectacular recoveries have been documented, it is not possible to demonstrate convincingly any favourable effect of corticosteroids, cytotoxic drugs or anticoagulants, used singly or in combination or in association with plasma exchange. As with most other forms of glomerulonephritis, carefully controlled therapeutic trials are needed. In view of the natural history of the condition, the use of potentially dangerous drugs can be justified only for those with a severe renal presentation and a marked abnormality on biopsy or for rapidly progressive nephritis. Therefore, therapy of Henoch–Schönlein nephritis is symptomatic. Patients with mild and moderate disease require no particular treatment. More severe disease will require measures for treatment of nephrotic syndrome or renal insufficiency and sometimes hypotensive drugs. Energetic symptomatic therapy is worthwhile because of the considerable potential for recovery from the nephritis. Relapses of the syndrome and of the nephritis sometimes occur at the time of an upper respiratory infection and regular follow-up is necessary until the urine deposit has disappeared. The appropriate duration of long-term follow-up is unknown; late-onset hypertension and renal failure may occur 5–10 years after the original illness.

Acknowledgement

I should like to thank Dr Margaret Chappell, Lecturer in Histopathology, Royal Free Hospital School of Medicine for providing the photomicrographs.

REFERENCES

1. Schönlein, J. L. (1832). In *Allgemeine und specielle Pathologie und Therapie*. C. Etlinger. Wurzburg, **2,** 68–70
2. Henoch, E. H. (1874). Uber eine eigenthümliche Form Von Purpura. *Berg. Klin. Wochnschr.,* **11,** 641
3. Henoch, E. H. (1895). Die hamorrhagische Diathese-Purpura. In *Vorlesungen uber Kinderkrankheiten*. Berlin, Hirschwald, **9,** 847
4. Heberden, W. (1800). Commentarii di Marlbaum. In *Historia et Curatoine*, Chapt. 78. (London: T. Payne)
5. Habib, R. and Cameron, J. S. (1982). Schönlein–Henoch purpura. In Bacon, P. A. and Hadler, N. M. (eds.) *The Kidney and Rheumatic Disease*, p. 178. (London: Butterworth Scientific)
6. Yoshikawa, N., Ito, H. and Matsuo. (1984). Henoch Schonlein nephritis: prognostic factors. In Brodehl, J., and Ehrich, J. H. H. (eds.) *Paediatric Nephrology*, pp. 226–229. (Berlin: Springer Verlag)
7. Allen, D. M., Diamond, L. K. and Howell, D. S. (1960). Anaphylactoid purpura in children (Schönlein–Henoch syndrome). *Am. J. Dis. Child.,* **99,** 833–855
8. Levy, M., Broyer, M., Arsan, A., Levy-Bentolila, D. and Habib, R. (1976). Glomerulonephrites du purpura rhumatoide chez l'enfant. Histoire naturelle et etude immunopathologique. In *Actualities Nephrologiques de L'Hopital Necker*. (Paris: Flammarion Medecine-Sciences)
9. Osler, W. (1914). Visceral lesions of purpura and allied conditions. *Br. Med. J.,* **1,** 517–525
10. Frank, E. (1915). Die essentielle Thombopenie. *Berl. Klin. Wochnschr.,* **52,** 454
11. Ackroyd, J. F. (1953). Allergic purpura due to foods, drugs and infections. *Am. J. Med.,* **14,** 605–632
12. Gairdner, D. (1948). The Schönlein–Henoch syndrome (Anaphylactoid purpura). *Q. J. Med.,* **17,** 95–122
13. Meadow, S. R., Glasgow, E. F., White, R. H. R., Moncrieff, M. W., Cameron,

J. S. and Ogg, C. S. (1972). Schönlein–Henoch nephritis. *Q. J. Med.*, **41**, 241–258
14. Ayoub, E. M. and Hoyer, J. (1969). Anaphylactoid purpura: streptococcal antibody titers and B_1-globulin levels. *J. Pediatr.*, **75**, 193–201
15. Pedersen, F. K. and Petersen, E. A. (1953). Varicella followed by glomerulonephritis. *Acta Paediatr. Scand.*, **64**, 886
16. Jiminez, E. L. and Darrington, H. J. (1968). Vaccination and Henoch–Schönlein purpura. *N. Engl. J. Med.*, **279**, 1171
17. Neiderhoff, H., Pernice, W. and Sedlacek, H. (1979). Purpura Schönlein–Henoch. *Deutsche Medizin Wochnshr.*, **104**, 1567
18. Liew, S. W. and Kessel, I. (1974). Mycoplasmal pneumonia preceding Henoch–Schlönlein purpura. *Arch. Dis. Child.*, **49**, 912
19. Sussman, M., Jones, J. H. and Almeida J. D. (1973). Deficiency of the second component of complement associated with anaphylactoid purpura and the presence of mycoplasma in the serum. *Clin. Exp. Immunol.*, **14**, 531–539
20. Cream, J. J., Gampel, J. M. and Peachy, R. D. G. (1970). Schlönlein–Henoch purpura in the adult. A study of 77 adults with anaphylactoid of Henoch–Schonlein purpura. *Q. J. Med.*, **39**, 461–484
21. Kauffmann, R. H., Hermann, W. and Meijer, C. J. L. M. (1980). Circulating IgA-immune complexes in Henoch–Schönlein purpura. A longitudinal study of their relationship to disease activity and vascular deposition of IgA. *Am. J. Med.*, **69**, 859–866
22. Cairns, S. A., Mallick, N. P. and Lawler, W. (1978). Squamous cell carcinoma of bronchus presenting with Henoch–Schlönlein purpura. *Br. Med. J.*, **2**, 474–475
23. Jones, N. F., Creamer, B. and Gimlette, T. M. D. (1966). Hypoproteinaemia in anaphylactoid purpura. *Br. Med. J.*, **11**, 1166–1168
24. Goldman, L. P. and Lindenberg, R. L. (1981). Henoch–Schönlein purpura. Gastrointestinal manifestations with endoscopic correlation. *Am. J. Gastroenterol.*, **75**, 357
25. Rodriguez-Erdman, F. and Levitan, R. (1968). Gastrointestinal and roentgenological manifestations of Henoch–Schönlein purpura. *Gastroenterology*, **54**, 260–264
26. Hurley, R. M. and Drummond, K. N. (1972). Anaphylactoid purpura nephritis: clinicopathological correlations. *J. Pediatr.*, **81**, 904
27. Koskimies, O., Rapola, J., Savilahta, E. and Vilska, J. (1974). Renal involvement: Schlönlein–Henoch purpura. *Acta Paediatr. Scand.*, **63**, 357–363
28. Greifer, I., Bernstein, J., Kikkawa, Y. and Edelmann, C. (1966). Histologic evidence of nephritis in patients with Schönlein–Henoch syndrome without clinical evidence of renal disease. In *3rd International Congress of Nephrology*, Abstract, p. 203, Washington
29. Chantler, C., Donckerwolcke, R. A., Brunner, F. P., Brynger, H. O. A., Gurland, H. G., Hathaway, R. A., Jacobs, C., Selwood, N. H. and Wing, A. J. (1977). Combined report on regular dialysis and transplantation of children in Europe. In Robinson, B. H. B. and Hawkins, J. B. *Proc. EDTA*, p. 77. (London: Pitman)
30. Counahan, R., Winterborn, M. H., White, R. H. R., Heaton, J. M., Meadow, S. R., Bluett, N. H., Swetschin, H., Cameron, J. S. and Chantler, C. (1977). Prognosis of Henoch–Schönlein nephritis in children. *Br. Med. J.*, **2**, 11–14
31. Kobayashi, O., Wada, H., Okawa, K. and Takeyama, I. (1977). Schönlein–Henoch's syndrome in children. In Berlyne, G. M. and Giavonetti, S. (eds) *Contr. Nephrol.*, Vol. 4, p. 48. (Basel: Karger)

32. Yoskikawa, N., White, R. H. R. and Cameron, A. H. (1981). Prognostic significance of the glomerular changes in Henoch–Schönlein nephritis. *Clin. Nephrol.*, **16,** 223–229
33. Heaton, J. M., Turner, D. R. and Cameron, J. S. (1977). Localization of glomerular deposits in Henoch–Schönlein nephritis. *Histopathology*, **1,** 93
34. Trygstad, C. W. and Stieham, E. (1971). Elevated serum IgA globulin in anaphylactoid purpura. *Paediatrics*, **47,** 1023–1028
35. Garcia-Fuentes, M., Chantler, C. and Williams. D. G. (1977). Cryoglobulinemia in Henoch–Schönlein purpura. *Br. Med. J.*, **2,** 163–165
36. Levinsky, R. J. and Barratt, T. M. (1979). IgA immune complexes in Henoch–Schönlein purpura. *Lancet*, **2,** 1100–1103
37. Hall, R. P., Lawley, R. J. and Heck, J. A. (1980). IgA-containing circulating immune complexes in dermatitis herpetiformis, Henloch–Schönlein purpura, sytemic lupus erythematosus and other diseases. *Clin. Exp. Immunol.*, **40,** 431–437
38. Coppo, R., Basolo, B. and Martina, G. (1982). Circulating immune complexes containing IgA, IgG and IgM in patients with primary IgA nephropathy and with Henoch–Schöenlein nephritis. Correlation with clinical and histologic signs of activity. *Clin. Nephrol.*, **18,** 230–239
39. Kauffmann, R. H., van Es, L. A. and Daha, M. R. (1981). The specific detection of IgA immune complexes. *J. Immunol. Meth.*, **40,** 117

INDEX

GPSR Compliance

The European Union's (EU) General Product Safety Regulation (GPSR) is a set of rules that requires consumer products to be safe and our obligations to ensure this.

If you have any concerns about our products, you can contact us on ProductSafety@springernature.com

In case Publisher is established outside the EU, the EU authorized representative is:

Springer Nature Customer Service Center GmbH
Europaplatz 3
69115 Heidelberg, Germany

Batch number: 10607224

Printed by Printforce, the Netherlands